SMILE...You're on
Candid Cancer

SMILE...You're on Candid Cancer

◆

My Picture of Life at its Best

Written by
John Wayne Warner
and
Georgetta Izora Warner

iUniverse, Inc.
New York Lincoln Shanghai

SMILE...You're on Candid Cancer
My Picture of Life at its Best

iUniverse books may be ordered through booksellers or by contacting:

iUniverse
2021 Pine Lake Road, Suite 100
Lincoln, NE 68512
www.iuniverse.com
1-800-Authors (1-800-288-4677)

ISBN-13: 978-0-595-40611-1 (pbk)
ISBN-13: 978-0-595-67819-8 (cloth)
ISBN-13: 978-0-595-84977-2 (ebk)
ISBN-10: 0-595-40611-4 (pbk)
ISBN-10: 0-595-67819-X (cloth)
ISBN-10: 0-595-84977-6 (ebk)

Printed in the United States of America

A Candle

A candle, when you first light it, is restless.
It weaves back and forth in all directions
like a grasping newborn child with no structure
purpose or direction.

As it begins to burn, the flame stretches for the sky
attempting to burn brighter and brighter.
Its light illuminates all around.

As it burns on, it dims jut a bit.
Then it seems to become very peaceful and steady
with no movement—as if its only purpose
is to produce light and become calm.

As the flame begins to go out, it becomes
restless and fights, knowing the end is near
by resisting with all its might to go on.

The inevitable happens.
The flame is doused with a small puff of smoke
which rises to the heavens
as a soul going to God.

By John W. Warner

This book is dedicated to John's family who has been there throughout his fight with their prayers, generosity, love and support.

We want to thank: Betty, for her many donations of food and trips into town; Sheryl, for her numerous hours of researching the internet and corresponding with medical experts on his behalf; Joe for his tireless trips to help with whatever needed to be done; John Sr., for his comforting phone calls and encouraging words.

Contents

Hi. My name is John Wayne Warner and I bet that you can guess who my namesake was. Anyhow, I was in law enforcement for more than twenty years until I was diagnosed with this disease. Prior to my illness, I was a pretty healthy guy, except for the poor eating habits, sporadic sleep patterns, and smoking routine; I guess I should say that, despite my habits, I was a pretty healthy guy. I made it through puberty, the Vietnam jungles and cancer. Well, I am determined to make it through that as well.

This writing covers approximately one year of my life, a mere season in the scope of anyone's days. Yet, this year has shaken and shocked me and brought me to my knees. It has reformed my thinking and altered my judgment of what really counts. I have come to understand what I can fix and what I must endure. To date, the chemotherapy and I have gone fourteen rounds with the cancer. I have continued to rally, but it has been a battle. In an effort to map out the sequence of events, the following pages include a synopsis of the time represented in this book. With that, I wish you good reading and I hope you enjoy it.

Timeline

John Wayne Warner

I. Testing to determine the cause of ongoing weakness, weight loss and treatment success.

A. *4/25/05: Appointment with general physician. Test: Urine culture. Results=negative*

B. *4/26/05: Ultrasound, Kidney. Results: negative*

C. *5/2/205: Bone Density Test. Results: normal*

D. *5/6/05: Colonoscopy. Results: negative for cancer*

E. *5/11/05: Endoscopy. Results: negative for cancer, Referred to Oncologist*

F. *5/18/05: CAT scan, Abdomen and Pelvis. Results: Lesions in the Liver*

G. *5/20/05: Chest x-ray. Results: negative for cancer*

H. *5/25/05: CAT scan—Chest. Results: normal x-ray*

I. *5/25/05: Nuclear Med., whole body scan. Results: Lesions in Liver*

J. *5/26/05: Blood work. Results: CA19-9=15,000*

K. *6/1/05: Cat Scan & Liver Biopsy. Results: Malignant lesions in the Liver*

L. *6/7/05: Blood work. Results: CA19-9=19,974*

M. *6/14/05: PET scan. Results: Multiple lesions in the Liver*

N. *6/15/05: Ultrasound. Results: Unremarkable*

O. *9/9/05: PET scan #2. Results: resolution of lesions in Liver. Necrotic tissue seen*

P. *9/13/05: Cat Scan, chest. Results: normal*

Q. *11/13/05: Ultrasound, legs. Results: no blockage or deep vein thrombosis*

R. *12/22/05: Cat Scan, chest. Results: some fluid in lungs and organ area*

S. *12/29/05: Cat Scan, chest. Results: Fluid retention drew out fluid. Neg. results*

T. *12/29/05: Ultrasound, abdomen. Results: some fluid retention*

U. *3/17/06: CAT scan. Results: compare to previous ct, tumors shrinking*

V. *5/2/06: PET scan. Results: one tumor in the liver, liver has decreased in size*

II. Chemotherapy and Blood work

A. *6/9/05: began oral chemotherapy cycle = every day for 2 wks. Off 1 wk.*

B. *6/9/05:Dr. Appt., Intravenous chemotherapy #1, round #1*

C. *6/16/05: Intravenous chemotherapy #2, round #1*

D. *6/29/05: Blood work. CA19-9=14,856*

E. *6/30/05:Dr. Appt., Intravenous chemotherapy #1, round #2*

F. *7/7/05: Intravenous chemotherapy #2, round #2*

G. *7/19/05: Blood work, CA19-9=2,198*

H. *7/21/05:Dr. Appt., Intravenous chemotherapy #1, round #3*

I. *7/286/05: Intravenous chemotherapy #2, round #3*

J. *8/9/05: Blood work + Red blood cell injection, CA19-9=555*

K. 8/11/05:Dr. Appt., Intravenous chemotherapy, #1, round 4

L. 8/18/05: Intravenous chemotherapy, #2, round 4

M. 8/31/05: Blood work, CA19-9=384

N. 9/1/05:Dr. Appt., Intravenous chemotherapy, #1, round #5

O. 9/8/05: Intravenous chemotherapy, #2, round #5

P. 9/13/05: Dr. Appt. Changed med for pain and nausea

Q. 9/20/05: Blood work, CA19-9=313

R. 9/22/05: Dr. Appt., Intravenous chemotherapy, #1, round #6

S. 9/29/05: Intravenous chemotherapy, #2, round #6

T. 10/11/05: Blood work, CA19-9=600

U. 10/13/05: Dr. Appt., intravenous chemotherapy #1, round #7

V. 10/20/05: Intravenous chemotherapy, #2, round #7

W. 11/3/05: Dr. Appt., Intravenous chemotherapy, #1, round #8

X. 11/10/05: Intravenous chemotherapy, #2, round #8

Y. 2 wks off chemo: 11/23/05:Dr. Appt. Intravenous chemotherapy, #1, round #9

Z. 11/30/05: Intravenous chemotherapy, #2, round #9: Blood work, CA19-9=389

AA. Ascities set in. 12/22/05: Dr. Appt. Intravenous chemotherapy #1, round #10

BB. 12/26/05: Blood work, CA19-9=2,305

CC. 12/29/05: Intravenous chemotherapy, #3, round #10

DD. 1/9/06: Blood work, CA19-9=9,994

EE. 1/12/06: began new oral chemotherapy cycle = every day for 2 wks. Off 1 wk.

FF. 1/12/06: Dr. Appt., began new chemo combination #1, round1

GG. 1/19/06: Chemo held. Low platelets: cyst examined

HH. 1/23/06: Blood work, CA19-9=2,634

II. 1/19/06, 1/20/06, 1/21/06, 1/22/06: White blood cell injections

JJ. 1/23/06 & 1/26/06: chemo held. Low platelets: Blood work, CA19-9=2,634

KK. 1/30/06: intravenous chemotherapy, # 1, round #2

LL. 1/31/06, 2/1/06, 2/3/06: White blood cell injections

MM. 2/6/06 & 2/9/06: chemo held. Low platelets

NN. 2/21/06: Blood work, CA19-9=351

OO. 2/27/06: back from cruise. Dr. Appt. intravenous chemotherapy #1, round#3

PP. 2/28/06: Dr. Appt. Port consultation for placement

QQ. 3/6/06: Dr. Appt. chemo held: Blood work, CA19-9=171

RR. 3/9/06: Port placement at hospital; 3/15/06: staples removed

SS. 3/17/06: intravenous chemotherapy #1, round #4

TT. 3/18/06: Red blood cell injection

UU. 3/18/06, 3/19/06, 3/20/06: White blood cell injections

VV. 3/24/06 & 3/28/06: chemo held. Low platelets

WW. 3/24/06: Red blood cell injection

XX. 4/5/06: Blood work, CA19-9=48, platelets=154

YY. 4/7/06 & 4/12/06: chemo held. Fatigue and good CA19-9 results, platelets=133

ZZ. 4/20/06: Blood work, CA19-9=33, platelets=127

AAA. 5/2/06: Dr. Appt. Chills, mood, weakness, Oral chemotherapy held 7 days, Antibiotic

BBB. 5/16/06: Dr. Appt. Ascities, fungal infection healed, Oral chemo resumed, CA19-9=77

III. Consultations with Cancer Specialists

A. 7/7/05: Cancer specialist, Good Samaritan Hospital, WPB, FL. Results: concurred with my oncologist

B. 8/2005: Sloan Kettering Hospital, NY. Sent pathology slides, referred with Drs. Results: concurred with my oncologist regarding treatment

C. 1/9/06: Miami Sylvester Cancer Clinic. Consultation with cancer specialist. Results: alternate treatment suggestions if/when the current treatment fails

Foreword

I have always had a good sense of humor. As a corrections officer, I have used that wit countless times to put people at ease. I resolved situations on a daily basis by utilizing public relations skills, verbal warning, and, occasionally, physical restraint. I have been trained to handle any problem that comes my way. I know what to do.

But, cancer is different. I find that I cannot talk it away. I can't use a taser to make it comply. I can't handcuff it or put it in a restraining chair when it gets in a rage. I can't even stop it with my 45. No level of force works with this disease. Cancer is a problem for which I am untrained, unprepared and shocked. Like most of you, I never thought this could happen to me. To battle this life-threatening menace, I am finding that it takes an ongoing regiment of drugs, chemotherapy, and a support system that has brought me to this place and time.

In the following pages, I have attempted to offer some insight gained through the day to day trials of my ten month and counting battle with this disease. This information is often given in a comical fashion because it helps me to laugh. God gave me this sense of humor and, apparently, cancer can't take it away. Having come up through the side streets of Indy, the jungles of Vietnam, and the settled, daily challenge of care, custody and control, I have now undertaken the greatest battle of all. I share my experience with you in hopes of providing something helpful and supportive in the process as I continue to fight. I have summed it up in this writing that I share.

Pass it On

I am what I am, working toward what I want to be
In the hope that I can bring joy, laughter, and help show as many people the correct path as I know it through this journey called life.

God has given me all that I need. Now it is up to me.
Oh…and now you. You're it. Pass it on.
Thanks, John

My friends, I truly hope that cancer never darkens your door. But, if
it does, I have discovered that you will need to learn humility, patience,
gratitude, and most of all, the ability to laugh to carry you through.
Oh, and one more thing…a backup set of clothes in the trunk of your
car.

Testing, 1. 2. 3.

✦

John's Chronicles

I learned many things in each day's battle. It began with the trips to determine why I had weight loss, fatigue and pain. This seemingly unending discovery process involved TESTS where I was slid, frozen, injected, poked, packed, punched, prodded, stuck, invaded and had pictures snapped of body parts that I didn't know I had. On top of that, I was asked some pretty silly questions including, "How are you feeling today?" when I looked thin and pale in an open-back gown. I was tempted to reply, "I think I'm dying, and how are you?", but I know that would not be kind, so I would normally just say, "Fine, and yourself?"

I've never been good at TESTS. In school, I failed almost every TEST that I took with the exception of the urine test. Still, they started in April and the TESTS continued with breakneck speed including urinalysis, ultrasound, bone density, chest x-ray, endoscopy, colonoscopy, liver biopsy, nuclear medicine body scan, catscan, petscan and more. Then, there was blood work and do they do blood work! I'm sure that they have more of my blood than I do. Soon they'll need a bigger refrigerator to hold it all. Of course, with all these tests, someone was bound to make a mistake, like when they informed me happily that I did not have uterine cancer (I am a man, by the way). I replied that I could have saved them the several hundred bucks for that diagnosis and, also by the way, I was not paying for that test. I will talk more about TESTS later.

Well, on to day two. Ha, ha. One of the most important things you learn is the difference between gas and diarrhea. Believe me, you'll only make that mistake once and you'll understand the reason for clothes in the trunk. But now to the annoying side effects of my intravenous chemotherapy, which are hiccups and itchy skin. These have been a particular nuisance during TESTS where you are instructed to remain still for several minutes or "we" (translation = I) will have to start over again. So, I would lie there aching to scratch the unexpected, rising itch washing over my nose while I tried not to let the hiccups escape. A tricky assignment, I must admit, but the freezer-like conditions in the hospital room did settle my hiccups after a while. It's a good thing that I like a challenge, I suppose. When I finally got home and told my wife, Georgetta, to cream me, she knew that I didn't mean to wipe me out. We were just trying to soak through the scales as each new skin layer came.

Then there is the contrast of the urine test and the ultrasound. Most people are familiar with these tests, but many of these invasions were new to me. Nonetheless, having had both now, I have noted some quirks. For the urine test they ask you to empty out and aim well into that tiny cup. For the ultrasound, they fill you with what seems like gallons of fluid, and then ask you to hold it while they press on your gut. They get you coming and going, from what I have seen.

At this point, I'm beginning to think that some techs just do that to watch you squirm. You couldn't do that job without getting a bit twisted I suppose.

Got Insurance

You quickly learn whether you have good insurance or not. To be sure, this realization is a shocking affair. Exhibit 1: After my first visit with the doctor, they gave us prescriptions and instructed us where to get them filled. The first oral chemotherapy drug was a two week supply. We waited the five minutes for the pharmacist to complete our order and I walked to the counter with my checkbook in hand. "That will be $900.00" the pharmacist offhandedly said while I made a great effort not to choke on my tongue! "What?" was all I could mumble before she explained that our insurance card wasn't valid now. When I got back my voice, I informed the druggist they would have to hold on to our pills. Then I walked weak-kneed from the drugstore to give benefits a call.

After procuring the newest prescription card, I was able to get the script for the standard $14 fee that we had always paid. But, it makes me wonder...what I would have done if the insurance didn't cover that $1800 a month and that was only one of the prescriptions I would need? No one likes it when I say this, but, after a couple weeks of that, I am thinking that a funeral wouldn't cost as much. Still, given a choice, I would rather have the meds.

The insurance companies, as well, are difficult at times. My wife Georgetta has dealt with them almost daily. Consequently, she has learned more than she ever wanted to know. For instance, the difference of one number in a procedure code can result in us receiving a $1,500 bill. An incorrect code, in fact, is the major reason for billing error and I am quite tired of hearing that a tumor marker blood test is "not consistent with the diagnosis". Translation, someone, somewhere between the doctor's office and the lab keeps writing the wrong code. I don't know who, but if and when I find out who is making our life so complicated, I may have to give them a piece of my mind!

In the Beginning

When I found out that I had cancer, the first thing I did was go into the bathroom and throw my blow dryer away. If I beat it, I would be happy to buy more combs and shiny new dryer, so its hair today, gone tomorrow, as far as I could see. Being a dabbler in the stock market, the second thing I did was buy stock in Kimberly-Clark (Kleenex), Johnson & Johnson (Band-Aid), Amgen (cancer pharmaceuticals), and Wyeth (Preparation H).

Seriously, that hot day in June, I learned that I had stage-four liver cancer that was metastasized from an unknown site. Because they could not find the primary, the cancer was officially termed Cholangio-carcinoma. When my doctor gave me the news, my questions were the same as everyone else. "How long do I have?", "Where does it go from here?" and, "What is the next stage?" He replied, as I remember, that I did not want to know. "Do we not have a stage one, two, and three?" I pressed on. "Yes", he said, "but you have already been through those." I was informed that without the Chemo, I could only have two weeks. With the Chemo, I could stretch that to four to five months. Now this sounded like a challenge and a worthwhile cause to fight for, so I took it on. Initially, I had no intention of taking Chemo from what I had heard about these dreaded drugs, but the time that he offered simply was not enough.

I was in uniform that day with full gun belt and duty gear. Can you imagine having to tell a stranger with a loaded gun that there isn't much you can do and that he has two weeks to five months tops? I do remember him telling me that I was taking this well. Looking back, I also recall the anxious expression on the doctor's face and I almost felt sorrier for him than for myself, except that, later that afternoon, I had to go home and tell my wife.

When treatments first begin, one usually knows little about cancer or the cures, except for the horror stories read or heard from friends. Consequently I didn't know what I was in for. My first go around with the IV chemo was a piece of cake. As a matter of fact, the first two months of chemo, which began in June of 2005, were no problem at all. I was even getting rather arrogant with my attitude because I was not sick and chemo seemed to be agreeing with me. My tumor markers, which are around 35 in the normal range, were nearly 20,000 when I first saw the oncologist. After the first few chemo treatments, those numbers had rapidly declined which meant that the treatments were working. By August, they were below 500 and I boldly told people that, after forty years of eight to twelve soft drinks and one to two packs of cigarettes per day, my stomach was now saying, "Hey this is nothing…bring it on." Like all of the other times when I have gotten arrogant about anything, I was soon to be shown the light.

The side effects of the undiagnosed cancer, as I stated earlier, were pain, weight loss and fatigue. After chemo began, there were the side effects of the drugs used to fight my disease. These varied with the treatments, but included pain, weight loss, fatigue, insomnia, hiccups, rashes, itchy skin, cracking skin, dry scaling skin, hair loss, numb hands and feet, fingernails and toenails turning dark and falling out, protruding, sore bones, ascities, teary eyes, runny nose, weakness, nausea, vomiting, mouth sores, headaches, dizziness, fuzzy feeling, blood vessels bursting in the eyes, constipation, diarrhea, hemorrhoids, loss of appetite, malnutrition, drop in white blood cells, drop in red blood cells, drop in platelets, and difficulty concentrating to name a few and there were a lot of shots. And by the way, *what did I mention the disease was again?*

Around August, three months into the combined chemo drugs, I began to undergo something new and strange. For the first few weeks, I didn't notice the time sequence, but after about a month, I started putting it together. I was getting the intravenous (IV) chemotherapy every Thursday for the first two weeks of each three-week cycle. On that third day, which was Sunday, I would invariably have to take to my bed. It was bad enough tackling the side effects one at a time. Now, I was getting an unsightly rash and nausea and weakness were all I could feel.

The only relief was to lie there and let the feeling take its course, which took until Wednesday, so I had one day before it started again and, need I mention that I really, really looked forward to Wednesdays? Soon, I also began to long for that whole third week simply because no IV = no yucky days. Nonetheless, while I lay there sick, in between having Georgetta at my every beck and call for something that I thought might help but did not, I isolated the symptoms and dubbed them collectively the *third day blahs*.

This continued until November when the drugs began to fail.

It's a Balancing Act

Around August, which was three months into the three week cycle of intravenous chemotherapy coupled with oral chemotherapy for two weeks, then one week off, I began to have many of the side effects. After giving it much thought, I've learned that it's all about balance, you see. The balance of meds and body functions was yet another continuing joyride on the cancer train. You would get everything going and working right with the meds you were on, then they'd throw in a new pill and the body would crash. For instance, you need pain pills, but they would cause you to be sluggish, so you would take over-the-counter meds to get things back on track. Then the oral chemo would kick in with its diarrhea side effect and whoo whoo...so you would have to readjust the meds engine day to day. Go, no go, go, no go...you get the picture. Well, the fun just never ends. The bright spot in all of this is that I'm still here riding the track, so it's all good to me. I'm not complaining mind you, merely pointing out the irony in the game.

Emotions also get out of balance when you are on the meds. Definitely, I find that I must use care regarding who I talk to and the subjects discussed. Some medications bring nerve endings to the surface of my skin and heighten my response to everyday events, like the effects my chemo is having that day. To give you an example, I have no problem discussing the pain of cancer, living, dying, side effects, or what will happen if I do not make it through. These topics are handled in a factual manner without feelings coming into play. But, tell me how much you love me, how much you want to help, or show me a kindness and the rollercoaster begins. So, I buckle up and hang on. It is often a bumpy ride while I try not to cry. Still, the feelings are strong and the tears often flow, which has never been like me at all. That is when I have to excuse myself, get a Kleenex and reinvent a cold. Crying, you see, just is not a guy thing.

That being said, friends and family tell me that I still make them laugh, so I guess some things do not change. That gives me pleasure, but I think it's no big deal since I've been doing it now for fifty years. By this time, it comes naturally and I should be good at something that I've practiced so long.

You must also balance the need to eat with the nausea that you feel and the up and down water gain with dehydration. Water pills helped drive off the fluid that the cancer/Chemo-produced water brought on. Then you had to take supplements that put the minerals back in that you just forced out. I know. It's confusing to me too. And ascities…oh yes, that swelling of feet, legs, tummy and other secret body parts. That is a story in itself.

In December, we took a quick Christmas trip to Indiana and Myrtle Beach at which point, I learned the new word called ascities. Let me tell you about ascities. It makes everything that you have **bigger**. Some might think this good, but trust me, it is not. Now, I cannot bend and touch my toes and this thing called IV chemotherapy is determined to show me what kind of deal it can be. Most mornings, when I get up, stand in front of the mirror and look at my stomach, I have the strongest urge to start humming my version of that old favorite song, "Havin' your baby. What a wonderful way of showin' how much I love you." Sometimes, I think water has taken over my insides. Just a consideration, but, if cancer can't swim, I'm in business because it has to be drowning in there. Come to think of it, I would much rather have someone tell me, "You're full of water." After all, I've been told enough that I'm full of other solid waste, which I am still trying to alleviate from myself.

Of late, my water gain has been fluctuating from day to day. This evening, it can be 128, only to have ballooned up to 131 the very next morning. It's yet another of the balancing acts to perform. "Up and down; Up and down. I'd like to get it all out, shut the door and lock it out forever." Oh well…

As the time goes by, my brain continues to flourish while my body says, "Karumbah! This is a lot harder than we thought." I look forward to rebuilding my body in hopes that I do better than I did it the first time around. Mentally, I think that I'm on track, no matter what the psychiatrists say. Kidding about that, but, a psychiatrist is about the only type of doctor that I haven't seen since this all began.

Upon reflection, I believe that ascites is my payback for all those jokes about women and their water weight gain. I'll never tell them again, I know that. After much practice of rolling to the floor from the sofa or my bed just to get on my knees, I have developed great empathy for the pregnant form. Sorry about the jokes. I just had no idea.

Once you have ascites, you will find that the job of, "putting on your socks" can be like squeezing ten pounds of sugar into a five-pound bag. Unless you've ever done this, I can hardly explain, but I will make an effort. Try this. Take your two thumbs and put them underneath your upper lip. Now, as quickly and forcibly as you can, pull it back over your head. Yell if it helps, but the key is, do not stop half way. Get the picture? That, my friends, is the *Compression Sock Shuffle*. After many tries and having the elastic snap against my skin, I invented this method to get my socks on.

Every morning, I would awake to new surprises as far as what body parts work, what hurts and where I cannot feel, and where new, developing lumps, sores, or rashes have formed. Each day is a different balancing act. I guess that makes life interesting. Yep, it's none of that same old, same old for me, so the adventure continues. About then, I realized that I wasn't as strong as I used to be. I could no longer lift, or fly, or jump mountain tops. It seems like just yesterday that was not a problem. But when I saw my wife carrying the heavy bags that I used to bring, it made me realize this change and it caused me to wonder…why hasn't she been doing this all along? Then I remembered that I didn't want her to. Anyway, so goes the battle, so goes the war.

Another landmark decision was to balance safety with desire, to swallow my pride and let someone else drive. I hated to give up that power that, as a law enforcement officer and driving instructor, I had treasured so. It's at times like these that you begin to realize how Miss Daisy felt. But bless Georgetta, who does not boast and humbly takes on her newfound role. My wife, I think I'll keep her.

I've found that cancer is devious and adaptive in many ways. It catches you off guard and changes from a creeping vine to a roaring lion in a single bound. Whether it is offering you those daily donations like hair globs in the sink or doubling you over with stomach cramps and swollen, sausage-like feet, you can expect it to be ever molding your shifting physique. Of late, I've been feeling like the Lone Ranger, traveling incognito through our town. Since I've dropped forty pounds and my features have changed, I run into people who don't know who I am. The only problem with that is I've known them for years and I do get tired of hearing, hi Georgie and…*who was that masked man?* Ah, but as soon as I begin speaking and telling jokes, they remember because the heart doesn't forget a joker or a friend.

Smoking

I stopped smoking cigarettes on January 1, 2006. I was motivated by the fact that everyone had been praying and helping wherever they could, so much so that I felt like a traitor when I took a puff. For a while during my illness, I justified smoking because it was truly something that I enjoyed, but that only lasted for a short period of time. I had smoked two packs a day for the last forty years. For that same forty years, people had been telling me that it was bad for my health. I used to reply, "By the time anything bad happens, advanced medicine will have come up with a cure, so I don't need to worry." Now, I am waiting anxiously for advanced medicine to catch up because I've got cancer with no cure in sight. I was so much smarter as a younger man.

For anyone trying to quit, here is some free advice. GET A HOBBY...My woodworking has been a great help during those sleepless nights. I can be sanding, painting, or waiting for polyurethane to dry instead of reaching for a cigarette butt. In addition, it is nice to have something to show for my work other than bad breath and money gone up in a puff of smoke. Friends and family seem to enjoy my craft gifts, but, who knows? They could be dumping them in the waste basket when they get back home. Even now that I have stopped, nothing upsets me more than an ex-smoker who, because he is miserable, is pestering others that they should quit. Besides, I know from experience that it does not work. So, I am going to leave you with a few thoughts. 1. I was very stupid to continue to smoke. 2. No one is as invincible as they would like to believe. 3. Even with this ongoing illness, I feel better now that I have quit and my bill for mouthwash has dropped considerably. I should have listened to them all!

Footnote: There are still days and moments when I think of grabbing a cigarette. For instance, after a meal or while driving with my window down, but I do not succumb. Lifelong habits are complicated and difficult to break. And, I would love to have all the money I have spent on cigarettes. Since I supported the tobacco company so very well all those years, it made perfect sense to me to write them when I got this illness and ask them for some help. Ha. Ha. But, do you know they ignored me and I was very put out, so now I have sold my tobacco stock.

The Unobtrusive Port

I couldn't tell my story without the mention of the unobtrusive little port that would set just under the skin so the doctors informed me. I initially resisted having the port, partly because I have managed to avoid surgery for 58 years and partly because I saw getting the port as resigning myself to the cancer or giving it a place in this war. Besides, the nurses told me that I had hoses for veins, so why did I need it, I reasoned with myself and I wasn't planning on taking Chemo long. As the skin got more sensitive and the shots began to hurt, though, I decided to make it easier on myself and the staff who often of late had to explore for a vein. O.U.C.H.

So I made my appointment and they inserted the *unobtrusive port* and covered their work with a lot of packing and gauze. I should have been tipped off when I saw the large bulge, but the soreness overrode my thoughts for the first few days. After all, as an officer my training when being wounded would be to strike back, so I guess it was a good thing they decided to put me out. Anyway, I was occupied with keeping the bandage dry during showers and protecting it while I slept. Then, they removed the bandage and the bulge appeared.

When I first mentioned the unobtrusive golf ball on my chest, Georgetta thought that was hilarious and that set me off. Then the nurses at Chemo heard about the unobtrusive softball and they laughed till they cried. As my audience expanded, so did the size of my unobtrusive port until it was the unobtrusive planet Pluto that sat on my chest. OK, so maybe it wasn't quite that big, but it appeared so to me when I looked in the mirror and I discovered my purpose was to make them laugh. It made others feel better and it helped me too. I guess the corrections officer is still trying to put people at ease.

In Search of Comfort

You know, cancer is pretty stupid because it kills itself. When you really think about it, either way, it will lose. In the meantime while I continue the fight, something else that has changed from the Chemo wars is my temperature. I've gone from being warm and needing the AC on, to freezing and wearing, multi-layered clothes. With a couple of layers, I look almost thin instead of emaciated.

It's not enough to need many layers, but each layer must be applied in a certain way. Only soft cotton can be next to my skin because I'm so sensitive that I can hardly stand to be touched. Sometimes, just to look at me hurts my skin. Besides, I don't really care for that unsightly rash.

I also need special bath towels and robes of micro fiber cotton and a cuddly blanket to keep me warm. Add to that cushy soft heel, elbow pads and white cotton gloves to complete the look and keep my fingers from cracking again. I look like the Pillsbury Doughboy, but I'm good to go.

My fingers and arms, well that's another tale. Georgetta has learned so much about nursing that she could get her degree. Coban for dressings that will not irritate, sterile, 2nd skin, Tegaderm, and adhesive; the bandage types just kept coming as she learned what to do. Eventually, she had so many dressings that she got a black bag. Now she is known as Doctor G.

Since I've lost so much weight, everything hurts including cushioned chairs and soft toilet seats. So I have a cushioned toilet seat for my cushioned toilet seat. And I have cushions of every shape and size along with goose down pillows and a goose down spread. Yes, only the softest 800-thread count cotton can be under me. My bank account is flattened, but I have a cushy bed.

I'm sure you have heard of the age-old connection between cops and donuts. I've always liked donuts. In the perilous world of law enforcement, I've learned that a good regimen of donuts gives you energy. Energy, in turn, helps you protect your behind. Well, now the word donut means an entirely different thing. It's still protecting my behind, but in an exciting, new way.

To ease my tender, swelling feet, we've tried every type of cushion that we could find including make-up pads, gel pads, bubble wrap, and cushioned padding from thick to thin. That led to house shoes of all colors and sizes, brown, black, navy blue, high tops, low backs, outside-the-house, and inside-the-house. They stand ready and waiting past the length of the bed. Does it ever end?

Then, we have heating devices, the hot water bottle, the standard heating pad, the moist/dry pad, the oversize pad, the electric throw, the full size blanket. Yes, we are prepared for the big chill here. I'm ready. I'm warm. With passion, I continue the fight.

Keeping on the Sunny Side

I am grateful for each new day. But, I am human too and sometimes I get sick and tired of being sick and tired. That said, however, I must confess some mysterious benefits to having a disease. When people learn the severe nature of your disease, friends, family and acquaintances alike will go out of their way to give you what you desire. For example, relatives bring food and, as a surprise, they buy you a cruise to simply be with you for that short period of time. People open stores early just for you when you ask from the door. You must be looking weak when people allow you to cut in line, and everyone generally tries to help you out. For an unkind person, these perks could be misused. I am careful, however, not to exploit these good folks and I believe my caution here is not without merit. If you take unfair advantage of this newfound power, look out...if the cancer doesn't kill you, the Chemo will have its shot, and, if you are too evil, and ask for too much...Who knows, the family might do you in. So, as you can see, caution must be used with this power. Don't Abuse.

Another odd benefit is with phone solicitors selling insurance. They only need to hear that you are definitely interested and could they come over today. "Did I mention I have Stage 4 cancer? So please hurry! Does that make a difference?" CLICK. They hung up. How ironic, when I didn't need insurance, they wanted to sell. Now that I need it, they change their mind.

Speaking of the telephone, everybody wants to call and see how you are. People that you haven't heard from in years call to ask about you when you are just wondering how they got your number at all. When you inquire about that, they relate that Frank told Hal who told Alice, etc. till it got down to them. The water cooler was busy that day, I guess.

One more perk is that anything you do garners compliments. Consequently, you think that you are the world's greatest artist, joke teller, and writer. All those nights of insomnia when you stayed up to create have resulted in many handmade gifts that you love to give. As friends gush about their beauty, you keep telling them that you don't make things…You make things better, but everyone thinks you are great. People stop telling you how to do things because suddenly, along with the illness, you have gained some knowledge that makes your art a masterpiece and every word golden. Here is my book to prove it, folks.

Bad tempered family and friends are changed by the disease as well. Like magic, they stop complaining when they realize their problems can't compare to my disease. Their two-hour wait at the doctor suddenly doesn't seem so bad and that is cool. And I must admit that I now share the need to appreciate more. Someone that I love used to tell me that we have to "stop and smell the roses" from time to time, to which I invariably responded "I don't have time to smell the roses because I plant the garden." Well, now I enjoy every whiff of my rose garden's scent and I've discovered that birds come to sing every morning in our front yard. Funny, but I never noticed that before. Guess I was too busy mowing the grass.

Translation Please

During my hospital adventures, I have discovered that doctors and nurses have a strange sense of humor and a secret code. Just to give you an idea, if a doctor says that you are going to feel a little pressure, hold on because it's going to hurt. If he says you'll notice some discomfort, look out…here comes a pretty good pain. If the doctor says this will probably hurt, then look for the exit and get ready to run because you will probably pass out if you don't get away.

Doctors seem to enjoy using specific words and numbers to classify pain, but they lose their sense of humor when you joke in return. For example, when they ask if you're allergic to anesthesia and you reply, "Yes. Every time that I take it, I just can't stay awake." Out of the blue, instead of laughing, the nurses want to stop everything and clarify. Go figure. Or when you joke with the anesthesiologist that you're a hemophiliac just before you pass out, they just don't get the jest. Medical professionals have a limited sense of humor, I've found.

They also use language that is hard to understand. You need the internet to translate the reports. Ascities, thrombosis, neuropathy, pleural effusion and such, these are only a few of their favorite words. Why can't they just tell us that neuropathy means numb? Are they afraid that we'll get too smart and try to take their jobs? I don't know, but my back is hurting from carrying that giant dictionary around.

Despite their obvious love of intricate words, medical professionals do understand the simple meaning of snacks. For instance, I have found that getting first class treatment in the doctor's office is fairly easy. It's a well kept secret that law enforcement officers are not the only professionals who love to eat donuts. Consequently, for the price of a dozen assorted, it is amazing how agreeable people can be from the secretaries and staff to the doctors, as well. The donut theory is proven over and over again and the results seldom vary; people work harder to get you in. But, I see the results as twofold. The translation here is a simple one and I don't need to search my dictionary to understand what it means. The sweet offering lets people know that they are appreciated and they, in turn, appreciate you. It's a win-win situation.

To Eat or Not To Eat

One of the major obstacles while taking chemotherapy is enhancing the ability and desire for food. I had to outsmart the nausea and continue to eat, even though I had little interest in nourishment. After all, I've always said that I wish they would make an all-nutrition pill that I could take once a day. I would take it for six days and eat lobster and shrimp on the seventh. In my healthier days, I ate to live. Even then, Georgetta had a list on the refrigerator titled *Things John Will Eat*. Now that I was full of a bevy of drugs, most foods that I ate had some nasty effects, as if my stomach took charge and developed a mind. "Chicken, no, don't want you. Get out of my house. Belly, run it on through" "Apples, not in this mouth. Back up you go. Bluuh."

I discovered Ensure which provided some nutrition and Georgetta gave me whole food vitamins and other nutritional supplements, but my taste buds changed like you change your socks. Pancakes that sounded delicious would no longer be appetizing after the ten minutes passed that it took to prepare them.

Another interesting effect of my evolving tastes were the cravings. Candy and sweets became my favorite foods. As my desires changed, I went through the donut, Twinkies, and cupcake stage. I would shortly move on to the jelly bean, starburst, lemon drop and skittle phase, which I am still in. Of late, I have added animal crackers and pretzels to my growing list. While I try to eat at least one meal a day that is often more of a challenge than I can handle, even though I know that I need it and it would probably make me feel better. Sometimes, it just doesn't sound or taste good. Because of this, I stopped going out to dinner since it seemed like such a waste, though I'm sure that Georgetta might prefer it at times.

Be it solid food or snacks, another problem with eating was processing it through. When the stomach allowed you to take it in, you then had the problem of where and how it would go. Personal questions suddenly become important. Did you 1 it or did you 2 it and if you 2'd it, what did it look like? Well, I have never had to describe how my bowel movements appeared. Come on! Is nothing private? Not only was it embarrassing, but it was difficult to explain: diarrhea, soft stool or *not like it used to be.*

And while we are on the subject, the bathroom now had a whole different importance in my life. While in my forties, I wrote a short story about people who read in the bathroom. My view was that the bathroom was an in and out place, rather than a place to loiter and read. And it used to be just that to me; a place that I went, stayed the necessary time, and got out. Now, I found myself spending long periods of time there, just hoping something would come out. On top of that, they would want me to describe what it looked like. Well, that's just another reason for me not to eat. Ok. Ok. I'll give it a try. Food, can't live with it, can't live without it.

Time

Time never stops
It just keeps on going
It runs like the river that never stops flowing
No matter what happens to you or me
Time never stops as you will see

I offhandedly wrote that poem when I was fifteen without any thought for what it might mean later in life. Back then, I was young and strong and full of myself. I remember saying right out loud, "I hope God takes me when I turn forty because a forty year old man can't do the things I want to do." For the past eighteen years, I have been thanking God for not listening to that foolish child.

Now I read that poem over and think of time. The concept of time, pre-cancer, can be verified by the fact that I used to wear a watch constantly to know what time it was. I was a busy man, always trying to run my efficient life. Time was a framework to get things done. Time was prioritized to important matters like keeping up with what was happening at work and listing what I must do to stay on track. All of this effort meant accomplishment and important promotions. The status they brought did feel good. I was driven with passion on top of my game.

Post-cancer time is a different matter. What I thought that I would never desire has now become fulfilling to me. For instance, I believed I would always work, at least part time, once I retired. Now, not having the pressures of work gives me quiet time to think, and I relish that.

Lately, I couldn't care less what time the clock says. All I want is to be awake with my wife. I have learned what is truly important and what will infinitely last…what is timeless, if you will.

As we reviewed this book for the millionth time, I got the feeling that we were having the most fun and just a wonderful time. Here, I must admit that we have also cried and been hurt as well and said things that we did not mean. I will say that these times have been easy to forget, and fewer than I even thought they would be.

Someone once asked me, "What does cancer do?" In its mildest form, it is certainly a thief of time, consuming the ins and outs of daily life, mostly revolving around the treating of the disease. That aside, the answer to that question will be different for everyone. There are factors like the type and progression of the tumor growth and whether it is you or a loved one who has the actual disease. While I have this illness, I have seen firsthand how my loved ones must bear it along with me.

First, my wife…you know the one who I said I would keep. Good choice on my part, I might add. Time, when I have down periods, is a struggle to her. Still, she is vigilant to care for my needs, often causing me to wonder where the strength comes from. Sometimes, I think that she is in more pain than I could endure. That is when I realize that she and my family are waging this war along with me. I know that I get sick and tired of being sick and I wonder at what point my family begins to feel as sick of it as I already am. I have tried to see that they get time away from this illness because it will wear you down.

You see, the time is easier on me because I have an advantage. If I hurt; they give me pills for relief, but the people who love me don't get anything to take for their pain. I guess this is where I come in, be it with jokes, attitude or just through comedy. I attempt to be their daily pain relief. Often, I know that I have just the right dose of *comedic meds*. But other times, I feel that I have fallen short. My medicating skills may not be exactly right, but I continue to try as long as I'm awake. In some ways, I believe this has brought my family closer, if by nothing more than to appreciate life. I know that I have a whole new understanding of that.

Now, I enjoy the small, but monumentally important things. Priorities have changed to what really counts. Love, home, family and friends have taken their place in the scheme of life. I am thankful for the gratitude and kindness of strangers. Georgetta always knew these truths of a meaningful life, but I am just beginning to understand. I value all of my family and friends and the kindness that they have shown Georgetta and me. I say this understanding the struggle of loved ones and friends when cancer strikes. They want so much to help, but they don't know exactly how. As your features change, it becomes more difficult. "You look good" comes from lips, but the eyes do not lie. In my pre-cancer days, I did the same thing. Now that I've been on the receiving end, I appreciate their love even more. Time spent in kindness is the timeless kind. Time here truly never stops.

Sarge

After six months of chemo, I had stopped going for walks in the evening with Georgetta. Energy, strength, and stamina can be drained by several types of disease. My ability to walk very far was greatly diminished by my loss of strength and weight. Finding problems a challenge as I do, I was searching for an answer when my sister, oh bless her, came along with a Segway human transport vehicle. Affectionately named Sarge, it made for a much easier and longer travel because Sarge did the work. It was a perfect solution, since a wheelchair was out of the question, but I needed to move. All I did was lean forward to go ahead, lean backward to reverse, use the handle to turn and try to slow down for Georgetta who was running behind. After some practice, we were ready to roll.

Tired but excited, Georgetta and I readied Sarge for our Island cruise. When the ship sailed into dock and they finally opened that awesome door, out we rolled. There we went, moving down the dockside, the island air blowing against our skin. Georgetta was doing a great job of jogging behind and Sarge was running smooth as butter. It was a beautiful thing!

What we didn't count on was the instant attraction that Sarge would incite. People swarmed around us like flies to ask questions and see a demonstration. "Is it easy to ride?" "Can you balance ok?" "Where can I get one?" The questions flew like arrows as tourists and islanders continued to encircle Sarge. Being the shy person that I am, I would normally never miss an opportunity to take the stage. However, I was beginning to feel uneasy with the constant crowd.

Sarge was so unique that we couldn't leave him parked for fear that a stranger would attempt to ride him or steal him away. I was glancing around when I saw them, the three large islanders with darting eyes. They kept looking from Sarge to my Chemo-wracked body and back to Sarge. I swear, I could hear their brains turning and I knew their thoughts, "I know I can take him and that Sarge would be mine." O.K., I was seeing that this was not good. In my healthier days, I could have taken on all of them, but now I'd do well to hurt those island flies buzzing over their heads. Still, my police training took over, so, Sarge, the wife and I were now standing guard.

We couldn't take Sarge inside, so we switched off going into the busy shops. Still, after another shop or two, with the ominous islanders getting ever more daring, we knew that it was only a matter of time before trouble would come. Being foreigners in foreign land, we decided to retire Sarge back to the ship. "At ease, soldier, you've pulled your hitch." "I guess you're just too special." was all I had to say. Too much fame, we decided, is not a good thing.

Life Changing Events

You may wonder why I treat the cancer with such a cavalier attitude. If you think about it, we all have cancer in one form or another…something physically or mentally eating away at us. You give it relevance or make the choice not to allow it to consume you or your thoughts. You judge the importance of whatever you are dealing with. Once you have done everything that you physically can, worry and thoughts of your problem have no place in your life. **I mean no place**. And I must add that you can't just talk the talk, but you must also walk the walk. People can tell whether you're sincere.

Has it changed my life? Absolutely! But, I prefer to look at what I have learned, instead of focusing on the pain and mental anguish that gives it the impact on our lives, as I have seen others do. If you want to talk about tragedy, you can go many places around the world and view catastrophic events including war, poverty, hunger, religious genocide, and travesties to children. Indeed, you can find disastrous situations at home, with mentally perverse adults who roam the streets of our cities and towns. In my opinion, these events are far more devastating than cancer, (no matter what the outcome). Thus, I refuse to give the disease the importance it seeks.

If you are looking for significant happenings, my marriage to Georgetta was a positive, life-changing event. Another meaningful time was my tour in Vietnam. This may seem like a negative event, but with any experience, I make the choice to remember difficult times in order to appreciate the richness of now. Cancer, on the other hand, is merely a bump that you can allow to defeat you or view as an experience that you will learn from.

Frankly, I am an experience man.

Speaking of experience, a recent life-changing event for me was writing *The Power of Words*. I wrote it several years ago for a group of officers that I was teaching for the Sheriff's Office Human Diversity class. At the time, I remember thinking, "Hey, this is good." and if people would use this, how much better family life, working conditions and everyday existence could be. Since I learned that I have cancer, it means even more. Next to family and friends, it has helped me gain perspective to fight this disease. Furthermore, it doesn't diminish my ability to make the world a better place.

I think back on the stories that we have all heard: about the man complaining he had no shoes until he saw a man who had no feet, or the person tired of looking at a filthy world until meeting the man who was blind. Once in my life, those were ready quotes, yet their unspoken meaning was lost. Now, I find it difficult to complain while I have the ability to make a choice on my own; I can make people miserable or make them laugh. The end result is simple. After all, it's easy to find someone who is worse off than I. Every morning, their names are published on the obituary page. Their time has passed, but mine is still here. I am inserting *The Power of Words* here because it helped me develop an optimistic way to find happiness with God, my wife, my family and friends. Please hold your applause until the end.

The Power of Words

I wish people could see what spews out of their mouths. Each time we talk, we fill the air with words and thoughts for all to hear. Think about what you have said today. Have your words taken flight and brought joy and laughter or made someone feel good with perhaps a compliment or have they been like arrows of complaints and gripes to do nothing by pierce the air and ears of those around you? Was the last person you talked to glad that you opened your mouth? Do they feel better for it or are they trying to defend themselves and clean up after the air that you have just fouled?

What do your words look like? Want to know? Just look in the faces of those around you. Are they happy—interested—longing for you to go on...or do they have that blank expression filled with a lack of interest? Must they defend against the arrows that you have directed their way?

The Power of Words
How many nice things have YOU said today?

You look very nice today	You are good
I love you	You work hard and I appreciate it
You are doing great	I will do what I can to help you
You do good work	Thank you
I want you to be happy	I appreciate you

Some comments can go for days without being uttered. In most cases, however, encouraging words should be spoken each day. Should you ever forget to give that "verbal hug" perhaps they will remember your kindness of the past and hold it as a cherished memory that warms the tired heart.

I have another idea that is deeply tied to *The Power of Words* which has changed my life. When it comes to cancer, I still hear people say, "Why me?" I have never heard anyone who just won the lottery speaking that way. No, they couldn't care less why the new wealth came. Just give them the money and they are off to go spend it. Well, I've been thinking about that a lot. I guess that I could say, "Why me?" and I'm on my way to try *to give a little back* for all the abundant blessings I've been given each day. The "What Can I Do for You" theory is an idea that has changed my thinking in a life altering way. I initially stumbled upon it while writing about ten years ago. Since I was dabbling in the stock market at the time, the concept of banking was fresh in my mind. This recent disease has only bolstered my theory to make it more common sense.

The theory goes like this. You see, I believe that we are all born millionaires and this wealth is kept in our *invisible bank*. Throughout our lifetime, we write checks and make deposits. As it happens, some people are overdrawn by the time they are teenagers or young adults. They make no deposits into their account or do not make enough to come close to the checks they have written. And deposits are so simple to our lifetime account—deeds of kindness, caring, unselfish acts, asking for nothing in return. These acts will build your bank account fast. Withdrawals, on the other hand, are careless, insensitive, self-centered actions, which we have all been guilty of.

When was the last time that you balanced the *invisible checkbook* you got at birth? After you do, if you have more than you started with, I would say that you are going in the right direction. However, some of you may find that your account has been closed. Well, don't panic. That is easy to fix. Look around you. Find someone to help; thank a person for their kindness; tell someone they look nice, you see what I mean. The only caution here is to be sincere. This should not be hard. Use the phone if you like, but make sure that your comments are genuine. There, your account has been reopened. Just remember, you are one million overdrawn, so let's get busy.

I also hear people saying that they want to know the secret of their purpose in life. Well, hold on! I have the long awaited answer that could change your thinking forever! You must strive to make an impact…have a mission to inspire. And, how will you do that, you may rightfully ask? In the spirit of the *Millionaire Birth Invisible Bank*, I say, do it through good deeds, encouragement, self-sacrifice and having high expectations to make the world a better place. Why? Just because you walked through it (not long ago, I would have said "ran through it" instead). It only makes sense that you give something back. By the way, this applies to all people, not just your friends. Indeed, the stranger is often the best person to help. Who knows, you may be an angel for someone and here's a shocker…You may end up helping someone that you thought you didn't even like. What a thought.

On a lighter note, other life-changing times to remember are these morning leg cramps. An alarm clock has nothing on these bothersome things. Here I am sound asleep and almost unconscious only to be awakened to 150% alert, trying to alleviate the cramps in the calves of my legs. I try every position including over my head. Still, nothing works and the muscles continue to contract. I know for certain that what happens in a matter of seconds in this excruciating pain really seems like days. Poor Georgetta rises early and is somewhere far away in the house, probably relishing the quiet, when she is suddenly alerted with a blood curdling scream that is my wake up call. Perhaps that is why she often tells me, "I feel your pain." This recurring experience is almost as eye opening as learning the difference between diarrhea and gas. I'm sure we both agree that we really need a better morning alarm.

Rambling Thoughts from Insomnia Central

After you have read this much of our adventure, you probably think that I don't know the meaning of irritability, except when I see it in others. Well, my friends, **you are right.** I am so glad that I have never been irritable! Of course, there are those occasional days when everyone in my whole world is wrong and I am the only one right. Hopefully, those days do not come often and, if I can recognize them early and keep them at bay…Right, if only it was that easy. This reminds me of the time my wife told me that I snore. Well, I don't think so. Just to prove my point, the very next night I stayed up all night and guess what? I did not snore once. You see, there are several ways to look at, judge, appreciate, or to merely agree or disagree on almost any matter.

By now, I am sure that you realize that I can be very difficult and, sometimes a regular pain in the butt. Hopefully, my good qualities, as few as they are, will overpower my faults. Just a note here to my wife and family: If my last statement is not true, you can go ahead and keep that to yourself, never to be discussed again, especially around me. Thanks, I needed that.

I am starting to feel a little pressure now because I fully expect McGraw Hill Publishing or, at least, Jay Leno or the Letterman Show to call and I feel that I have so far to go with my book. When it's finished, I believe I'll have the makings of a first class movie. I think George Clooney should play my part. What? Well…if you can stop laughing long enough, I will continue on. Did I mention delusional as one of the side effects of the medication? Oh well, I'm sure that I told Harvey…you know, the six foot rabbit sitting right next to me. No, I am not crazy and I don't see things that are not there, but as you can clearly see, I don't like to discuss topics that put me ill at ease. Now that I have gotten that out, I will discuss this illness, living, dying, and pain. I am willing to discuss these serious matters, as well as silly subjects, while the latter, to be sure, is where my talent in misdirection is best applied. Remember, irritability is how we began this conversation.

I have had a lot of time to think in the last year and when I write that all of my thoughts have been positive, I don't simply mean that I think that I am going to win my war with cancer. This disease has opened my eyes to some very important facts. I truly feel that I have won already, if only because I know now that time is the only thing that continues on. Yeah, yeah, I know that you have heard this before. Our mortal bodies do not continue, although we think that they will, hope that they will, and truly believe that they will. The truth is…They don't! I am thankful to the cancer for what it has caused me to see and I would take it again if it would benefit those that I love. No truer words have been spoken.

In the last year, I have tried not to use my cancer as an excuse and I hope that my family and loved ones will do the same. You know what I mean, "I'm not going to work today because I'm so upset over my (insert relative here)'s cancer. I have never been much on excuses. Besides, all the time and effort spent weeping will not bring us one bit closer to a cure than they already are. You can take as many days off from your obligation as you will and I'll still be where I am right now. We are all doing what we can to help, and the rest is up to God, the doctors and me. So, PLEASE, if you need an excuse to do something that you know you shouldn't do, use the war or the starving children overseas. Both of those causes are more important and fixable than I from your place in the scheme. Also, I am *not* fighting this fight so that you can damage yourself in my name. OK, I am officially off my soapbox. Sorry, but I just had to get that out. Ahhhhh…I feel so much better now.

With all this contemplation, I have also observed, listened and learned and I now see my family in a new and different light. You see, some of my faults can be explained. I hate to admit it, but I come from a broken home. Yes, my parents were divorced. I believe that I was almost forty at the time, but such traumatic events are hard to overcome. Or, we could go the jail route; I've been in and out of jail on a daily basis for the last twenty years. I am to the point where the state of Florida pays me monthly NOT to come back. After all, twenty years as a corrections officer and you deserve something in exchange. Then, there is my mother who in the past year has resorted to staying all night with men for ten dollars an hour. Well…she is eighty years old and the man is ninety-seven, can't get out of bed and needs to have someone there all night, but that is beside the point. I am still traumatized. (In case you haven't guessed, she was a companion). Now we add to that, my father is the world's greatest entre-*manure*. I will say no more. Except for my sister…well she got all the brains and my brother scarfed up the ability away from all of us. And, what did I end up with, but this struggling humor to help me overcome. So perhaps you can see why I am like I am. I think this would be a good time to state that all the opinions and statements are from the author's perspective and not necessarily shared by the publisher, A.B.C., N.B.C., my family or any of those guys.

Seriously, I have researched my cancer extensively. I have also talked to cancer survivors. I have <u>not</u> spoken with anyone who lost their fight against cancer, but that is for another day, I believe. In the meantime, I know that my cancer is not something you can see or touch. You can, however, see the results of the cancer and chemo. This may be good, but I just don't know. What I do know is that the lost weight, weakness, and pale coloring that you can see are bad enough. It's not something you can hide for long. All the jokes, laughter, and great mood will not disguise how you look, so you should tell your loved ones as soon as you can handle it. That is one thing I learned.

Another vital bit of information is to trust your doctor. You and your family should trust the medical staff. If you don't have faith in them, how can you beat the disease? In my opinion, you can't. So, if you don't trust them, find someone that you will have confidence in. Faith, you know, though a mere five letters, can cure, save, move mountains and change worlds, and, most important, put you closer with your creator, no matter what your belief. I don't think that I have ever met an atheist, but I do know that in all my years I have never heard anyone thank an atheist for some good fortune they have had.

Addressing the cancer, I don't know what brought it on and I only want to look to the future, rather than the past. Researchers state, however, that diet, smoking, and stress all have something to do with disease. As soon as I win this war, I can take on the how and why to see if I can make a difference for others down the road. For now, I choose to help people through lowering stress. It is a fact that laughing takes your mind off the negative thoughts of the day and, who knows? Through your efforts you may be someone's *Saving Grace, All Purpose, Stress Reduction Friend*. Even better, you may be saving their life by keeping them from getting sick. By the way, if you do try this theory, stay away from my wife's ex-husband. He plainly needs too much help…ha, ha. Seriously speaking of making a difference, have you helped someone today with a smile or kind word? Well, read *The Power of Words* one more time, oh, and thank you very much.

As far back as I can remember I have taken great pleasure from making people laugh and smile. I have learned to refine this method to make sure that the humor is at my cost and not that of someone else, and not hurtful to one person while funny to another. I am sure there are times when I fail at that lofty goal, but I am getting better. Cancer, now that I don't mind offending, or even killing off. As a matter of fact, that is what this book is about, though I occasionally wander off topic. These modest side trips on this adventure are good for me, however, and hopefully provide some insight as to how I feel.

I haven't talked much about dying. Perhaps because I am so focused on living and fighting the sickness and on what I need to do that it just doesn't come up. Also, I have Georgetta set up with retirement, insurance and a modest income, so that gives me peace. If I don't win this battle, that will be the first day of the rest of my eternal life God willing.

While I have no trouble talking about the cancer, living, and dying, I have had a real problem for the last few years with people telling me that they lost their wife a year ago or they lost their husband recently. Every time that I hear the term "lost" my natural response is "Well, tell me where you last saw them and I'll help you bring them back." It sounds as though they have misplaced their loved one, not that the loved one has died. Apparently, some people have a major problem with merely stating that out loud. I am not trying to be funny here or make anyone feel bad. I guess I just want to understand.

Speaking of feeling bad, I sometimes have guilt because I *don't* have any pressing problems to deal with. My attitude is positive…I have the attitude of gratitude. I often ponder that if scientists could develop a non-narcotic pill for attitude, they could lessen the need for all other drugs and cures for disease. In my opinion, those pills should be free or at least dirt cheap. Most of the time, when you see how much your medication costs, that alone will make you sick. Come to think of it, have you seen the price of land lately? Even dirt, now, is not cheap.

Oh, there's one pressing problem that I forgot to tell you about. Lately, I've been thinking a lot about initials. That's right. I don't know what it is with initials, your own and your loved ones as well. You want to put them on everything. I don't know whether you think people will forget you if you don't make it or you just perceive that your initials, (JWW, in my case) are special and signing every sheet of toilet paper will be of some value to someone who works at the wastewater treatment plant. I don't know if you think that your loved ones will forget their own initials, GIW, if you don't have them written on enough knick knacks or what. You think it is necessary at the time. Oh well. The initials, JWW, are easy to spell and, in most cases, there are only three letters to worry about.

Got sleep? NO!!! It seems that when you are sick or in pain, this would be the time to sleep and when you feel better, this is logically when you should be awake. It's a great theory, but in real life, thoughts and feel-good times are not that often and they come at times like 1 a.m., 2 a.m., 3 a.m., etc. in the wee hours, the more wee the better, it would appear. And who do you share this with when the rest of the world is out like a light? That is where I should be right about now, ah but, no such luck for me. Oh well, as long as I am getting better and becoming less of a burden on myself and those I love.

During this road to recovery, I have seen many positive changes in family and friends. Now, I hope my loved ones will go back to focusing on their own lives instead of trying to help me. It has been great, by the way, and hopefully we won't forget the knowledge of the experience we have all gained. I know that I have learned much. I'm excited to put all these years of writing into practice…good ideas I've been told many times. Yet, I don't really feel that I've used my writings to their full potential. Besides, I have a lot of ground to cover telling people the secret. Come on, you remember…. *The secret to make people laugh*. It's now 4:30 a.m. How many people do you think I could make laugh over the telephone right this minute? Now, that would be a challenge for sure.

After reading this over, I can see that I should have been in bed a while ago. I seem to be rambling, but the later it gets, the more wonderful my writing seems. Funny, but from 1:00 a.m. to 3:30 a.m., everything I write does look and sound great...I mean the best! From 5:00 a.m. on, the same writing doesn't seem nearly as good. But, it's late. Soon, my wife will be rising to tell me that I need my rest, the birds will be singing, and I will be snoring away. Ha. Ha. Incidentally, I tested myself again last night to be sure and I DO NOT SNORE. Good night and sweet dreams. JWW

Life by the Numbers

Well, the day that was coming since I was told almost a year ago that I have cancer, is here. On this day, April 12, 2006, my CA19-9 (a tumor marker that helps indicate cancer cells) is officially down to a reasonable level. In June 2005, the number was an astronomical 19,974. {The normal range is 25-37.} I was at 14,856 after the first treatments, then all the way down to 313 in September 2005. Then the tumor marker numbers began to fluctuate and rise. By the end of December, it was back up to 2305. By January 2006, it had climbed to 9,994. This meant that the treatments had stopped working. So, in January 2006 we began a new treatment plan with two new drugs.

Since my numbers have continued to decrease to an ALMOST NORMAL 48, but what does that mean? I should be jumping for joy and screaming knowing that I will beat this disease. However, right now, I'm more concerned with the people that I need to help than with what *my numbers* are. For months, we have lived by these numbers, built our lives and our plans around them every day. So, I am indeed happy, in fact overjoyed that my numbers are almost in line. The doctors say that it means the treatment to this point is successful. But does that mean I can stop? No answer there. Doctors would probably not say that. After all, what would happen if they recommended ceasing treatment and the cancer returned? Perhaps, I am pondering, it is not even gone…merely lurking in some crevice, biding its time.

I have found that cancer is a patient disease and chameleon-like in its attack. No, I hold no trust in those sneaky cancer cells. They are able to transform and overcome because the secret of cancer is to have control. Happily for me, I'm a control freak too, so the conflict rages on. About now, though, it appears that I have taken charge.

Still, I look back at this struggle with the cancer and realize how important "numbers" have become. Along with the tumor markers, there are a multitude of *counters* that gauge your success in this cancer war. You have electrolyte counts that need to be adjusted when you have water weight gain. Gatorade, magnesium, salt intake and that sugar I love, these and other factors come into play. Then you have white blood cells counts that drop from the IV chemo and leave you disposed to infections. Often shots will correct this, but even that takes some time.

Feeling weary? That might be your red blood count numbers crashing down to the ground. Well, let's get another shot to alleviate that. Then, there are liver function panels that must be taken into account. These, my friends, are only a few of the numbers that cancer affects. And, lest I forget, there are the numbers of the dollars that it takes to keep battling this war—for prescriptions, treatments, day to day medical needs, and ongoing tests to determine your state of health. Unfortunately, they have no such test to keep track of you state of mind with these numbers, numbers, numbers that are pressing on your brain. That is why I have given that job to my wonderful wife. Whew...Now I can get back to the cancer war.

We saw the oncologist recently since my tumor markers have gone down. "Does this mean I am cured?" "Can I now stop taking the chemo drug?" "Am I now less than a stage 4?" These were some of the questions I was bursting to ask. The response that I got was less than I had hoped for. I learned that the cancer was being held in check, but not cured and that I would need to continue the chemo drug. "Well, he is a good doctor...but he's not our primary physician" was what I had to say.

But, please don't misunderstand me. I am glad for the numbers to help us keep track and I am especially happy for the number 48!!! Still, I have much to do. Rather than numbers, it is times in my life that made me happiest; times when I brought joy to those around me. One event happened recently when I passed out one of my handmade *appreciation* cards while checking out at our local store. The young, clearly pregnant lady who received it had been very polite and I wanted to show her how grateful I was. I gave it, saying "Read this when you get the chance." and headed to the car while my wife finished with the check-out.

I was just opening my car door when I heard her yell "Thank you", looked up and saw the young woman standing on the sidewalk and blowing me a kiss. Apparently, when she read it, she was visibly moved because she immediately left her station where Georgetta was waiting to be checked out and sought me out before going back to her work. She then shared with my wife what a rough day she was having. "Yesterday", she spoke with emotion, "I buried a friend." "Your husband made my day." "He was sent from God."

My wife relayed the message when she came out. The feeling it gave me is hard to explain. One thing I realized is that we often cannot know what a kindness means to others. Sometimes, it is little, yet, at other times, with the smallest concern, you can touch someone's world. It brought me great joy to have been a small part of making her smile. To me, that was an unforgettable event. Memorable moments, not numbers, make life worthwhile. By the way, we have provided *appreciation* cards for you to pass out. They are located in the back of this book.

Bad Days, Bad Weeks and Whatever

And the battle goes on. As my numbers continue to move in the right direction, my body is telling me a different story. I often hurt more and keep losing weight. I can't help asking if I am getting so much better, then why I feel so much worse. The answers I obtain are somewhat satisfying which include an explanation of how my body is struggling with the disease and the medicine I am on. Still, I want to know, **is this as good as I am ever going to feel?** For these types of questions, no one has a response, yet the answer, I have discovered, is in one word of the question itself. *Feel. Do I feel? Yes! Yes! Yes!* Well, as long as I continue to feel *anything*, then I must believe that I am going in the right direction. Not being able to feel would mean that I have lost our greatest emotion which is caring. The ability to love, desire, be happy or sad and have compassion for others means that I am winning this game. Maybe someone should write a song and call it feelings or go back to the 60's and 70's and get the score written by Morris Kaiserman (aka Morris Albert) instead. Perhaps Shakespeare should have said "to feel or not to feel" instead of that phase about being in his memorable Hamlet soliloquy. I think it would sound even better. Oh well, just a thought, another 2 a.m. inspiration.

Despite the numbers, anyone with cancer will have bad days and weeks and whatever. What do I mean by that? Well, the cancer markers aside, I am weak and tired and the side effects of the medicine are a constant matter to deal with each day. *Bad days*...I have had a few, sometimes I think a few is wishful thinking on my part. As I have said,

I have no problem with dying if this cancer takes a turn, but I want to know where I stand. If that happens, I need to know when the time comes, not because of anything I did or didn't say to my family or even last words that I need to express. I have done that already. I just want to prepare them and make them all laugh one more time.

Really, there is nothing left to say. They all know how much I love them, especially my wife. I try to express my gratitude and love every day and I worry about her with this heavy burden that she and the rest of my family carry. My wife is the one who hasn't had a break for the past year or so.

During the bad days, your spouse has the most influence to pull you along. No matter what happens, she smiles and says, "That's ok." "It's no big deal." "As long as you are here, I'm doing great." "It's not a problem that you burned down the house." "We can always get another one." or "I wanted to move anyway. This was a good thing." I have spilled, broken, torn and made numerous messes that she has had to clean up, not to mention waiting on me head to toe. I say head to toe because from my hair to my shoes and socks and all in between, she has worked on it all at one time or another. If it's not getting me to doctor appointments or patching me up, she's getting me all straightened so I don't look like a fool. She is there. I love you Georgetta.

Getting back to the bad days, with a great support system, you can get through anything, and mine happens to be the best; thank you Georgetta, Sheryl, Joe, Betty and John. To all the others, I have not forgotten you at all. I just don't have enough pages in this book to mention Georgetta's family, mine and Georgetta's work family and friends, and all of their contacts who have held me in prayer. From the bottom of my heart, I thank you for helping me stand up to this disease and beat it down. THANKS, I NEEDED THAT. Where have I heard that before?

You will find a *Thanks, I Needed That* card in the back of this book. If you make copies and just pass out one or two a week, what kind of change do you think might take place? You have already bought this book. Why not let it work for you. Who knows what you might receive in return beyond a great feeling about yourself. And the person that you have given the card to…you have certainly added to their day. If you like my positive attitude and want to feel this way, this is a place to begin. Thankfully, you don't have to get cancer to open your eyes or clear your mind. I have already done that and I would not lie to you. Besides, I want nothing from you but a smile. I can't make you monetarily rich or solve all your problems, but I can tell you truthfully that laughing and making others feel good is a far greater wealth, and it has taken the edge off any problem that I have ever come across.

The Gifts of Cancer

This may not sound reasonable to you, but, believe me when I say that I have received more from my cancer than it has taken from me. Even if it eventually takes my life, I still win by virtue of the knowledge that I have gained. Several of those *gifts* are listed here.

My new outlook is probably the most important gift that having cancer has produced because I now have a stronger urge to help others. This desire is not limited to dealing with cancer, but branches to the issues of life itself. Our concerns are most important to us. Be it the car, the kids, money or a loved one's health, all these issues are relevant because they are ours. But when you try to help others with their problems, the strangest thing happens; your troubles get smaller, or perhaps you don't think about them nearly as much. I'm not sure how the change comes about, but I know that it works.

I have also learned how to *really* value time. Two years ago, if you asked me what I wanted from life and how I was going to get it, I could have gone on for hours explaining what it was and how hard work and keeping my eyes on the goal was going to ensure the results I desired. However, my desires have changed. Daily plans that once had great importance now seem less relevant to me. Nonetheless, these issues deserve some thought and work. I still need to care for my wife financially, but I don't have to make these issues the center of our world. As long as she has food, clothing, shelter and a steady income, she will be fine and we can focus on time spent together. If you ask me now what I want out of life, I would tell you that I have it all and I need nothing material to feel that I am a success. My efforts today are spent on giving back and bringing others into that ever-expanding circle to do the same.

What you say and what it says about you, these are vital elements of character that I have learned of late. Over the years, I discovered how words, though they may be in the form of an offhanded remark, have the ability to hurt those we love. Because of this understanding, I have learned to use care not to cause hurt feelings or emotional harm. With the advent of cancer, however, I've rediscovered how my words can also uplift and heal. I realize how much I appreciate the kind words of others. This makes me want to give that feeling back and the pleasure it gives me is a wonderful thing.

Having cancer has helped me to understand love. The word has perhaps had more definitions and verses written about it than any other word in the dictionary. Those definitions and writings are different because each of us thinks in individual ways. Some believe that you need two people to experience love while others would say that an unselfish feeling towards someone would describe it well. My definition of love is the way my wife, family and friends have treated me over the years, particularly since I became ill with this disease. If not for God and their care, I would not be here now. You see, I know how it feels to receive love and hope and pray that I succeed in showing that feeling to others as well. Love is something that you give that has no beginning and no end because we keep the circle growing. We give love in truth and hope that we are worthy to get it back.

Finally, I feel very strongly that I have something left to do in this world. I am not quite sure what my great mission is yet, but making you feel better or giving thought to others may be the right track to that mysterious goal. Indeed, we are all so blessed in this life that we can always find someone who is worse off than we are, no matter what our circumstances. The crafts and poems I have made or written and given away have brought people joy while they gave me the feeling of a job well done. However, I have received more joy in the giving than the people who have received the gifts.

Faith

Now to the chapter of our book that brings everything together…Faith. This means different things to different people. I accept as true that everybody makes a choice to believe in something, even if it's not to believe. As for me, I do believe in God and hope that he believes in me enough to forgive me because only he can. I also give him credit for anything good that I have ever done or said. I truly am not capable of anything without him. I sincerely feel that on the day I was born, God gave me that *Million Dollar Invisible Checking Account* I discussed earlier in the book, meaning everything I need to do good and make it through this journey we call life. I can't think of another thing to say except thank you, thank you, thank you.

I know that we all need help from time to time, but that's just for insignificant items that more money, more work, or simply trying harder can bring. There is a saying that if money can solve your problems, you really don't have any…but merely an inconvenience. Money cannot make you well or smart or a better person. You and God can accomplish these tasks however, *and it's absolutely free!*

I have seen and experienced so many miracles in my life that it would be impossible for me to not believe in God. I do need to say that I have not always felt this way and up until about seventeen years ago, my actions were not something to be proud of. This faith that I've begun has been growing all these years, not just since I have been sick. As a matter of fact, some of my writings are as much as thirty-five years old. I guess what I am trying to say is that I don't believe that I have ever been an evil person, but I have committed my share of sins and perhaps enough for two or three other people as well.

Back to faith, I would not be here today without the strength of the wife and family that God has given me. God only knows good, love, compassion, fairness, and forgiveness…How could you not believe in a doctrine like that? Indeed, this book is inspired by God and if you think differently after reading this far, well, you probably missed a lot of what it is all about and should read it again. Better yet, you should give this book to someone else and buy another copy for yourself. Maybe the second time with a new book will do the trick; I know it will help my book sales! And who knows, the person you give the book to might love it or just like it. If it helps even one person, it's a success as far as I am concerned.

Well, I have said everything at this time that I wish to say about…what was that disease we were talking about? Oh, cancer, that's right. Sometimes, it just slips my mind. There are so many important things going on in the world. If you did enjoy this book and want to know if there will be a book two, the answer is yes! Look for either Laugh Your Cancer out of Your Body or My Picture of Cancer Never Developed by John W. Warner or My Husband's Lost Battle with Cancer by Georgetta Warner. Also, if you have experienced cancer and would like to talk about it, that would be welcome and appreciated. In the meantime, **God Bless You**, whether you want it or not. The End…*But Not Really.*

Concluding Remarks

It is now eleven months since I began this fight. Today was one of those days that followed another sleepless night, so I slept during the day. It is late and I have a doctor's appointment tomorrow at 9 a.m., so I guess I should try to get some rest. I am sure that tomorrow will be chemo day. After that, it will be two weeks of trying to eat and sleep and build up my blood and platelet count. Staying over one hundred on platelets seems to be the magic number. I think this might be a good place to end my book and take care of more important matters; cancer, family, loved ones and paying off bills. I feel like I have a really good handle on the cancer, so I will continue to make use of my talents, whatever they may be, the best way that I can.

After writing this book, I realized that my foreword, though honest at the time, was not accurate regarding my not being trained for this situation. I was wrong. I have been training all of my life for dealing with this. Attitude, state of mind, vision, foresight, and my policy of always having a backup plan have aided greatly in this war.

I also learned from this writing process. I was trying to decide who this work has helped more, my loving wife or my family and friends. Then I realized that the obvious answer is me. I've learned more about myself, my capabilities, and how I'm still acquiring the knowledge to put them to use. I also understand how this book can offer promise in other situations, not necessarily pertaining to a terminal disease. And, if my theory of survival is right, I will let you know in my sequel.

I have learned that with any disease, the more attention that you give it, the more important it becomes. If a fireman were focused only on the fire, he would never save the baby. So, I won't give this malignancy credence while I beat it down.

According to the doctors, I am doing well. Four to five months has stretched into the better part of a year and counting and I continue to manage the chemo pain. Meanwhile, when someone thinks of me and breaks out in a smile or they chuckle and grin, I feel joy. It's not that I have done anything great, but the happiness that I have helped produce is not forgotten and thus, neither am I.

For the most part, I am pleased. My attitude remains focused on getting well, rather than falling into the *why me* zone. It is where I am going that counts while I am here on this earth. When my wife came and said to me, "SMILE, you're on Candid Cancer..." I did my best to describe the struggles of this disease. And, generally, I've done it with a joyous heart. Now my writing is finished, but my journey continues. After all, there are still people out there that I haven't made smile.

Now, I am tossing the ball into your court. Yes, you guessed it, Tag, you're it. So go out there folks and make the world a better place. Give some comfort where there is pain. Offer friendship, love, and abundant hugs and try to make someone laugh because laughter truly is good like a medicine. In my opinion, it's the best medicine of all. JWW

Another Point of View

✦

Georgetta's Account

I do not have my husband's gift of wit, so if you are looking for humor, go back to page one. I do, however, share his positive outlook on life, Christian values, and ideals. Together we have worked hard for the past sixteen years, often holding two or more jobs each and striving for the retirement dream. We were almost there. We had managed to set up a plan to retire. In less than a year, we were preparing to buy a motor home and travel the country. That was before the curtain fell. Now, I often wish that I could turn back the clock.

When a loved one has cancer, they suffer a great deal. That is the understatement of the century. Words cannot describe the pain that my husband has endured with a smile on his face. I have watched and nursed him every day. I have seen him change from the strong, handsome man that I married to a man who struggles to sit, stand, lie down and walk, depending on the illness and side effects of the drugs he is on. I have watched him bent in agony with stomach cramps, too sick to eat from the IV drugs. I have seen his body shrink while his legs and feet ballooned. Too many nights, I have reached in the darkness to feel his heart. Through all of this, what I have not seen is John give in.

What I have seen is a courageous, grateful man who is giving to others from the crafts he has made. In wonder, I watch this man that I married, excited to continue with kindly deeds. Every day, I wake to a man who is thankful for days and hours and minutes of time with never a question about why he was given this frightful disease. Nor can I ask this question because I know that each breath is in God's hands.

What I Have Learned

I have learned much from the way John has worn this disease. You can get an indication from our earlier words. He is beating it down, as he loves to say, but that cancer, as well, packs a very strong punch. While the fierce war continues, my heart presses down. My grandfather battled cancer when I was 18. I took him to doctors and chemo, then radiation later on. He was strong like my Johnny and I admire that. In many ways, they were similar, I'm beginning to see. I've learned that strength of character separates this type of man.

I have also learned that I have weakness to deal with here. This was all unexpected, as it always is, and I find myself struggling to deal with the pain. There is no way to tell you how deeply I feel, but I shove the tears down to stay strong for John. That is something he has taught me. No matter how hard, you must press on. Though I am sure it is with much effort, it appears natural for him because he has such a presence of strength. The only way I can do that is to look past the disease that lives on his skin and see the resolve in his beautiful heart. That gives me courage to help my John.

Another thing I have learned is that we are on God's plan and schedule rather than our own. This has taught me patience as day to day he leads us. When extraordinarily difficult situations arise and you feel as though you can't go on, that is precisely the moment, if you let him, when God steps in. I say if you let him because God will not enter the picture unless you invite him in. If we open ourselves up to him, he is faithful to provide the hope that we need to maintain. In my lifetime, I have found that the harder a situation is the closer God holds us in his arms. Certainly, you can *see* his handiwork in the world in the trees, the flowers, the singing birds and the magnificent ocean two miles from our door, just to mention a few. Yet, if you close your eyes and let your spiritual self feel, you will *sense* his presence as well. He is waiting to come at the perfect place and time. So fear not, as Jesus and his angels say in the Bible. And what is there to fear, after all?

Love in All Its Forms

Since the first time I met him, John has been the light of my life. The struggles of time have only brought us closer together. I realize that John is my blessing from God sent to heal me from a troubled past. For as long as I remember, it has been Johnny and me. We are a team, united through the good times and bad. It is no different with this illness.

Love can mean friendship. When I learned that John had cancer, I could not take it in. With all these years together (sixteen married plus nine as best friends) I have married my best friend. Yet, he is so much more. He is part of the breath that I draw every day. For all this time until now, when something hurts, I would bring it to John. He always fixed it or made it all right. He has the art of attention, taking in my words like a starving man. I feel important when I talk to John. I know it is selfish to feel this way, but whenever God takes him, be it soon or many years ahead, I know that I'll never be special to anyone again. Yet I will hold the blessing of being truly loved.

Love is so much more than the first, romantic kind. Granted, that is usually how it begins. Yet, when illness strikes and those desires can no longer be fulfilled, it is by no means the end of love. Love, in true form, is a feeling between man and woman that cannot be lost or taken away. It cannot be diminished with the beating of time. When you really love, a mere hug can heal. Just the sound of his voice, this is love to me.

Life is change, I heard someone say and I used to wonder what that could mean. Since I was a youngster, I have hated change. Perhaps it began when I started first grade and had to leave my sick father who passed on when I was ten. I could have stopped it. I could have helped him. I could have kept him alive. Those were thoughts I had when my dad went away. But I have learned from John how to suffer change. He calls it adventure that he relishes in. Because of my husband, I have learned to trust that, while life is ever evolving, love stays the same.

Love in its essence assumes many forms. People often ask now how I am. My response is always the same, "As long as John is here, I am doing well."

Insomnia...From My Side of the Bed

Some things do not change. One of those habits is the way that John sleeps. Rather, I should put it, the way he doesn't sleep. Insomnia has been a problem in our house for years. John worked on third shift for two and one half years before he became ill and his sleeping patterns have only gotten worse with the disease. It's not unusual to find him wide awake and creating at 3:00 A.M. or periodically napping on the sofa when he finally wears down while I get up every few minutes to see if he is ok.

The next morning, he will sleep in, but I cannot regimen myself to staying in bed. By 7:00, I am up and moving since morning is my productive time. Of course, a few days of this deprivation makes for one tired wife. Without my needed sleep, I go around yawning all day while John is asking, "Are you tired my love?" "Why don't you go take a nap?" Oh, if life were that simple. I can't sleep during the day.

I've thought of methods to help him rest at night including not taking a nap during the day, giving him warm milk before bedtime, a warm soak in the tub, and going to bed at a regular time. He just lies there for hours trying to sleep. But, you give him a shot at that bed after he's been up all night and it's a different story. Then he suffers from creative exhaustion, I suppose, because he's out like a light before his head hits the bed. He barely gets covered before he's gone, snoring logs to the ceiling and back.

I've tried staying up with him at night, but I can't keep from nodding off any better than he can sleep, so it looks like we have a problem here. So far, nothing has worked to get him sleeping *regular nights*, so I'm thinking of giving him a curfew to bed. Ha. Ha. And, I am beginning to wonder about this vampire-like custom. If he starts nibbling my neck, I don't know what I'll do! Seriously, I don't know what I'll do if I can't start getting some important R.E.M. sleep! Oh, to sleep, perchance to dream (Sorry for the plagiarism, Will).

Seriously, I know that John needs rest now more than ever to fight his disease. While he does sleep during the day, I wonder if it makes up for the loss at night. When he was younger, he regularly kept late hours, but sooner or later, this will wear him down. So, I continue the search for a way to get him genuine rest. Our latest attempt was to purchase a lush recliner chair thinking the comfort would help him relax and he would be more ready for bed. I'll have to let you know about the results of that experiment as the jury is still out.

Nonetheless, he comes each morning from insomnia-land laden with work. Obviously, John's creative genius peaks late at night. For instance, just this morning around 5:00 A.M., he was showing me pages of fresh written thoughts and a couple of crafts he was working on. Now, at that time, my productive motors are just sliding into gear, so, of course, I took the pages and began to type them in. Suddenly, I realized how well this works. He is black to my white, yin to my yang. Come to think of it, John and I remind me of that poem about Jack Sprat. Remember, he could eat no fat and his wife could eat no lean, so between the both of them, they licked the platter clean. Yes, it all works out fine if it weren't for that pesky need to sleep. Yawn, oh well, Yawn. Sorry, I dozed off. Yes, back to work.

Transitions

I take this man to love and to cherish, for better or worse, in sickness and in health…I gladly took those vows many years ago, never dreaming that sickness would visit so soon. Yet, change, I have found, is a part of life. Despite my dislike for it, it still comes. Now, because of the cancer, our lives have been greatly altered. Where it used to be common to jump in the car with a moment's notice and be off to the store, now we have to prepare for even a trip to the bank. Since John is often tired from the months of chemo, it takes longer to get ready for a shorter stay. Pleasure outings are scrapped or put on hold and we have learned to relegate time to important trips. Only vital travel, such as a testing and doctor's appointments, becomes a sure thing. This is fine with me. Personally, I would rather be home with John.

Another transition was from walking to taking Sarge. Thank God for Sarge. What a cool, smart-looking machine for my very cool guy. It took a bit of getting used to, but he has become a welcome part of the family. Now, we continue our evening walks. Soon, I will be riding my bicycle to put me on even keel with John and Sarge. Once we get our new pattern set, what a team we will be.

When I look around, our house appears the same. The furniture we purchased over the years together remains intact. We still live in the apartment we bought after months of searching to find just the right place. On the surface, all seems well. Yet, with my new vision, I see that much has changed in our somber house. Oh, John still laughs at times, but it often has a hollow ring. I feel the great burden he is trying to hide. I sense the pain in his beautiful face. What I would give to draw that away; to take it on myself, so that John could fight his battle with less of the sting. Vietnam, I am satisfied, could be no worse than now. My love thought himself finished with horrible war when he left Vietnam.

The sofa where we sat and snuggled to watch comedy on T.V. is now my haven alone. John no longer sees television as important in the scope of his days. Nor do I really, yet it provides me some semblance of normalcy. Somehow, it helps me feel that all is right in my fantasyland and my husband isn't sick in the room next to me. Laughing at a silly sitcom character makes me think of pre-cancer John. For this space in time, I can remember moments when he made me smile, or played a joke with that mischievous twinkle that he gets in his eye, or loved me in some special way that touched my heart. For a while, I can think about that vacation out west or some other plans we often talked about instead of the chemo appointment he has next week.

Oh, to have that time back with my John. But, he is correct that time never stops and where it has gone, I cannot conceive. Where it is going, I often do not wish to know. So, I hold onto faith and do not think about it while I sit and remember my strong, virile husband coming through our front door and holding me close to make everything right. For now, I wish he could fix the creeping monster that lives in his flesh; crush it and yank it all out, then throw it over the highest cliff and return to me as he was before.

With all the struggles that live in my heart, still I always consider how we've been blessed these few short years. Love that is genuine is a truly rare gift and I look forward with hope to many more days with John. In the meantime, I know he is trying. When I look at my husband, I continue to see his smile and his hopeful eyes. In those blue-green pools that remind me of a soft, dewy morning in a fertile dale, my Johnny lives on.

Make 'Em Laugh

What can I say about John's humor? Make 'em laugh. John must have been born with that intrinsic theme. Laughter swells with every beat of his heart, it is so engrained in the vital core of who he is and what he is driven by. John without laughter is like a day without song, the sun without the moon, me without him in my life everyday. That and his charm are how he won me...along with his incredibly cute butt. I won him, by the way, through picking the beans from his chili, but that is a story for another place and time.

His humor is legend with family and friends. His jokes are constant, unforgettable, successful, and thoroughly planned. Yes, John has been the bright spot of countless peoples' days for many, many years. And a well-orchestrated joke is a beautiful thing-an outlet for stress, a pleasing experience, and a joy for all...*most of the time.* On rare occasions, I must admit that he has gone too far. How you may ask can a joke go awry? Well, it happens when the enthusiastic joker has *priorities that are meaningful only to him.* What could I mean by that odd little phrase? Well, let's begin with the shopping cart.

It happened one sunny afternoon at the grocery store when John and I were running in to pick up some food. We were rushing to get to another date, so I grabbed the cart quickly, rolled it to produce, and turned to grab bananas with one hand while I held the cart with the other. Clink! Clink! "What was that?" I asked jerking around toward the unfamiliar cold, heavy pressure that was set on my wrist. "You cuffed me!" I stammered, looking down at the cuffs hooked, one on my wrist and the other fastened to the handle of the shopping cart.

"Get this off", I continued in a barely controlled voice while he stood there laughing like a hyena cub. "Get this off…NOW" I repeated as patrons walked past us in wonder, probably thinking I was some criminal caught in the shoplifting act. At least, that is where my mind was at the time.

"Ok, Ok." he finally replied when he had calmed down enough from his belly laughs. After an eternity, he reached for the key. That's when I remember thinking it would be over soon and I was finally beginning to calm myself down. But that was before John informed me that he had forgotten the key!! FORGOTTEN THE KEY!!! He remembered the joke, he remembered the cuffs, he remembered to laugh, but he FORGOT THE KEY! "Don't panic" he said calmly, "I'll pick the lock." Then totally unruffled, he went digging through his jeans. After a moment, he smiled and pulled out a paperclip. So, I stood there, trying to cover my shameful *incarceration* with the side of my purse while people passed, gazing at my husband poking the lock on his joking cuffs. And, being an officer he had, of course, brought the official cuffs; Nothing but the best for my John, no sir.

After a few minutes, his smile wasn't so wide, and I could see that he was having trouble releasing the lock. I had visions of my arm hanging out of the car window, still hooked to this cart from our moving car. Oh, my. I was feeling faint. "If I have to walk through checkout hooked to these cuffs, YOU WILL GET TO EXPLAIN HOW THEY GOT ON MY ARM." I was speaking from panic mode now, partly in fear that he wouldn't get them off and partly terrified of what story he might invent at the checkout line if he did not. After all, he was riding a euphoric, joke high by this time. With his stand-up comic mind, there was just no telling what he might say.

"Hold still." "Calm down, I will get it" was all he would tell me, and he did, after several long minutes of embarrassing attention from the gawking crowd. Well, that was just an *adventure* as John loves to say, and it gave him a story to share at work which he did, rest assured, with many laughing results. So memorable was that image and his blow by blow account that people from work still mention it today. But, in my humble opinion, *he had gone too far.*

It Sounds Like a Challenge to Me

To say that John loves a challenge is a gross understatement. Part of his constitutional makeup is his love of competition. When he gets up each day and I say good morning, he often responds, "That sounds like a challenge to me." Often this challenge fetish has been quite extreme. Still, that trait has aided him in this battle with which he is engaged.

And, how would I know that John loves a challenge, you may want to know. I have seen it firsthand. I recall many times when he carefully laid plans to reciprocate for some joke that was played. John relished the opportunity to show who actually ruled in the *Joking Challenge* game. I am here to attest that the ruler is John. After all, if you spent the time working toward that goal, you, too, could compete at master rank.

When I think of John's zest for a challenge over the years, there is one adventure that stands out in my mind. *The First Date* was an ultimate test of his skills. It began at his job where John was a star of the joking challenge. Ultimately, he would win in the end. Everyone knew that...except for Dennis. He was stubborn, I suppose, and determined to play the bigger joke.

It began with small jokes that kept growing until John decided to win the game. Dennis had mentioned having a first date that evening. In passing, he told someone where he would be. John patiently waited until evening. Then, he had a friend drive by to be sure Dennis was there. That friend called John when Dennis went into the restroom and John called the sports bar where the starry-eyed couple was having their meal.

"This is Dr. Wengate," he informed the bartender. "I am looking for a man named Dennis." "Dennis. Is there a Dennis in here?" the bartender yelled across the room. "Not here" the bartender answered when he got no response. Dennis could hear his name being called from the restroom. He was trying to hurry to see what was going on.

"I know he's there...," the "Doctor" continued. "His wife is in labor. He needs to get here NOW!" Well, the bartender, upset now, yelled loud as he could, "Dennis, GET TO THE HOSPITAL. YOUR WIFE IS IN LABOR. GET TO THE HOSPITAL NOW!" Oh dear, but the girlfriend got angry and left while Dennis sat in shock from his favorite stall. The conclusion to it all...that was the last time he tried to top John.

John has been through many challenges in his life and has written about several of these experiences in this book. Perhaps they have made his cancer easier to bear. I cannot say, but I do know that John has been a phenomenal example for me. I have seen how he smiles when I know he was feeling very ill and I have witnessed the gratitude in their eyes and the smiles of appreciation on each face. Somehow, it means so much when a person who is obviously ill makes an attempt to help others when they could use help themselves. More times than I can count since John was diagnosed with this disease, I have heard him offer to help others when he barely could walk from fatigue.

A challenge...Yes, John understands a challenge; that much I can guarantee. As with every other instance, he has taken this on full throttle.

Take Your Time...Hurry Up

That is a phrase that John has planted and set to root in my head by repeating it over and over again when he was ready to get going somewhere. He called it a joke every time. Personally, thinking back on it, I call it brainwashing instead. Nonetheless, those words are so intrinsically implanted in my mind that all he needs to say now is, "Take your time" and I immediately translate it as, "Hurry up." Even when he says, "I really mean it. Take your time" it doesn't mean a thing. Nothing pipes into my head except "hurry up, hurry up, and hurry up." Thank you very much John.

How did he accomplish this feat? It took several months, but, as usual, he was a diligent man. When we were getting ready to go out, he would always say loudly, "Take your time." followed immediately with a suggestive whisper of "Hurry up." With enough repetition, it is now as natural as taking a breath. When *anyone* utters the words "Take your time." all I can think is to get on the move. My perception is permanently altered. Thank you ever so very much John.

Really, knowing my husband, I could expect no less than to hurry up because that is what he has always done. The first day I met him at his restaurant, Deli-mans, he was moving swiftly, rushing from the video games to the tables to the kitchen in back. In fact, I soon learned how much he loved to live fast which is the opposite of how I believe one should live. On occasion, I would like to slow down and enjoy the view instead of seeing the Grand Canyon at 90 miles an hour while John points out fading sights as we go speeding by. "Look Georgetta! There's a bear. Never mind. It's gone." "Quick, it's a deer. Oh, you missed it." Are you beginning to see what I mean? After all, we had to get to everything, so one grows accustomed to living with glimpses of life.

From what I understand, he even has people at work acclimated to his *Take Your Time* theory. Apparently, he has used it in abundance with his daily work, while giving jail tours, and at the firearms range where he used to instruct. They tell me that if you say "Take your time" at the range, someone will invariably finish the phrase, "hurry up." Yes, my husband is a success in the brainwashing game. How many lives he has touched…and *trained* along the way.

To be sure, John always knew how to get things done. He took two giant strides for each footstep that most people make; he was in such a hurry to finish a task. Still, once that task was completed, we were far too busy rushing to the next *big thrill* to enjoy the success that we had just attained. Life in race mode was exciting and never dull but, it left me exhausted at the end of a day. I've often thought that John was trying to cram many days of living into every hour, sort of like his *Compression Sock Shuffle* applied to his life. But that is John.

Now, all of the rushing has come to a screeching halt since John became ill. That familiar running has become a memory of the distant past, but rest assured that John is still moving along. His type of movement is all that has changed. Now, he is waging a *mental war* with this cancer through his power of will. Yes, he continues taking chemo and the other medicines have helped as well, but his determination is as strong a medicine as any pill that he puts in his mouth. While the cancer does its worst, I can still hear John saying that he is beating it down. As he continues to profess against it and will it to leave, I can almost hear him saying, "Take your time." *"HURRY UP!!!"* "Take your time." *"HURRY UP!!!"* and I know that my John is still a diligent man.

We Are Family

We are Family...Do you remember the song? Those few words encompass so much. Most of the time, being part of a family is wonderful. At other times, the individual and collective needs of its members can be part of the trial that each family goes through when a crisis comes.

From time to time, people get short with each other once nerves become frayed. Families are no different. In fact, they are often more inclined to be caught in the storm of the struggle *because* they are close. Objectivity, I have found, is lost in such times as these. Because we are all individuals, we handle emotional pain in our own unique ways. Some cry at the merest whisper that John is having a bad day while others choose to search for a new way to help. Some find misdirection; joking or not keeping contact at all is a way to endure the hurt.

Other means of helping are abundant as well. Some people feel that they can feed the cancer away or lessen the reality of the moment with whatever skill they possess like running errands, sending get well cards, dressing a wound, doing laundry, or fixing a sprung door. Of course, saying a prayer is at the top of that list and rightfully so, as far as I am concerned. Regardless of the assistance offered, it is each person's attempt to express their concern and help to ease the loved one's pain. These heartfelt endeavors bring both the giver and receiver emotional ease. Grave illness, I have discovered, stirs the need for fellowship in family and friends.

There are times when the sickness gets even to John. When this happens, he doesn't want to get out of bed and he gets emotional quite easily. These are the times when I feel the most helpless. The most I can do is try to make him comfortable and share with him when he wants to talk. He once said during a difficult time that he wanted to go to sleep and wake up and this would only be a nightmare he had. That pretty well speaks to how we both feel. Still, the nightmare continues.

The majority of the time, I control how I let myself think about this illness and what it is doing to John. I shut off negative thinking when it tries to get in. There are times, however, when the pain bares heavy and lies hard on my chest, so much that I feel I can't breathe. When that happens, I pray and envision that hurt in a big metal pail. I give it to God and he provides me with peace and strength in return. The Bible says to cast your cares upon him and I have never failed to see that truth come to pass.

What Is Special about John?

Special is such an all purpose word used to describe many types of people. It can mean anything from wonderful to horribly mean. When most of John's friends and co-workers call him *special*, it is with the best regard for his humorous, positive ways. A few, however, use more unique terms. For example, his supervisor has called John an enigma for years. To answer that calling, John began saying that his supervisor thinks of him in a religious way; he thinks that John is his cross to bear. Another friend refers to my husband as *unique* all the time. While each of his colleagues has their particular fashion of explaining John, they are all really saying how extraordinary he is. After mulling this over a while, I can now shed some light on the *special* traits that make John stand out.

You know, people always say that they love John, but.... This sentence is inevitably followed with a series of explanations. For instance, "but I couldn't ride in a car very long with him" or "I couldn't put up with the practical jokes." In fact, for years now, when I meet John's co-workers, they will undoubtedly grab my hand or give me a hug as if they know me well. Then, their eyes will gloss over and a wave of sympathy will spread across their face. "Oh! *You are Georgetta*", they will say. "You must be an angel" or "You must be a saint" or "God bless you, dear."

Well, the blessings are great and I can certainly use all the good wishes that I can inspire. Still, I fail to understand their responses and have often been puzzled by their sympathetic gaze. They must not care for excitement, I have come to decide. As for myself, I believe excitement is good and it always takes place in surroundings where I feel entirely safe.

John is simply a fun-loving guy. When he has a feel-good day, he is ready to roll. He wants to embrace that sensation till it dissolves away and he likes to accomplish that doing different things. After all, who wants to stick to the same old routine like always driving the speed limit or having *regular* sleep? And, as John loves to say, if you stopped for every one of those red lights, you would never get anywhere. Even now, when he doesn't feel like driving and has to give me the wheel, he compensates by telling me where to turn and the places to stop. Yes, I like adventure and its middle name is John.

I will admit that John has a unique way of looking at things and perhaps that has affected me some. For example, when he had ascities on his legs and I was putting on cream and he said, "Whatever you do, DO NOT let your fingernails touch my skin!" Well, some might have been offended and said do it yourself, but I understood that his legs hurt and my fingernails felt more like rakes on his aching flesh. So, I found it hilarious that he put it that way and of course, I was careful applying the cream.

John is not only fun-loving, but he is funny as well. I could offer countless examples were you here to converse. Since I am limited by the space of a page, here is one of late that first comes to mind. It was the time when we tried using an athletic supporter to keep the ascities from swelling his groin area again. When the device would not fit, John's immediate response was "Well, I know one thing...I'm taking *all* of the department and my family too when I go to the store for an EXTRA LARGE." Most people would be upset with the growing pain, but not John. No, he finds humor in everything and that humor is stronger than any pain. His instantaneous reaction is to make me laugh. That, my friends, makes John a special man.

John has always been an entertainer in his exceptional way and he uses that ability to bring people cheer. It's a remarkable talent that he has just recently seen as the great gift it is. But he is so much more than a joker because that trait is connected to John's giving heart. I have witnessed this characteristic on occasion through the years when we were both busy with careers, but never more than since he has been diagnosed with cancer.

This disease has turned him into a driven man. When I first met John, I knew his power of persuasion. During all our years together, I have witnessed his power to persevere, his honesty, his passion and drive. Indeed, he has always had these qualities of leadership. The only thing changed with the advent of cancer is the focus of that God given power. Keeping busy with training and running his shift has been replaced with the need to give something back for the blessings that John recognizes he has received. He does this with gifts he has carefully made and encouraging words to the fellow patients and staff at the doctor's office, the hospital, and the lab to draw blood. He does it with donuts and humor that brightens a day and puts people at ease. He does it with appreciation cards and jokes to make them smile. He does it with offers to lend a helping hand and with the words he has set in this book. The methods vary, but the results are the same; John gives of himself to lift his fellow man. If his podium could be large enough, he would lift up the world.

You may think I am prejudiced where my husband is concerned and you would be correct in that belief. But, the words that I write are true. The results are factual and the desire to repay is a very real feeling that comes from his heart. Do I think my husband is *special?* You bet I do! No matter what happens with this cancer, the love he is showing can't be taken away. His hope is to start a chain reaction of kindness and hope and, you know…it is working. *It is spreading every day* and will continue to sweep the nation, one heart at a time. Why, you may ask? Because each person is endowed with special talents and the ability to make the world a better place. So, John plants the seeds and God waters the garden and makes it grow.

One simple, yet profound concept that I am reminded of by my *special* husband is that, though kindness is a small thing, small things can make a big difference in the world. John doesn't just say it...he lives his faith every day and God sustains him to continue in hope. I'll be right there, too, touching hearts, making up the cards, typing the pages, laminating his art and rubbing the cream without "touching my nails on his skin."

Amazing Grace and a Smile

We first learn about life from our parents. Mine were each talented in particular ways. My mother was a hardworking woman born into difficult times who worked in restaurants most of her life. Perhaps that is why she was stubborn and set in her beliefs. You might think of that as a negative trait and it often could be; I certainly would have attested so in my teenage years. But that willful nature has seen her through many hard times with diabetes, two bouts with cancer, four amputations in a four-month hospital stay, and a bevy of other health issues. Her favorite phrase has to be, "I'm not going until God is ready to take me home." No matter what happened, she would never give up. From my mother, I learned determination.

My father was a woodcrafter, photographer, harpist, police officer, minister and a farmer, though not all at the same time. I learned much from this versatile man. As I helped him meticulously plant the garden, I learned how to wait. When we reaped the harvest, I came to understand hope and the value of planting a seed. His abundant kindness helped me know how to give. Yet, the greatest gift from my father was teaching me faith, an endowment that continues to grow exponentially. With each new struggle, I rely on it more.

Because of what I have learned, I receive each morning with gratitude and hope, knowing we are not promised to always be healthy, happy or well-to-do. We are assured, however, the strength to endure any struggle while considering that trials are what make us grow. If I had no sorrow, I could not fully appreciate the joy that I have with John. Nor could I get up tomorrow and relish moments while I help him through this complex time instead of focusing on the pain in his walk and the struggle in his eyes. Because of determined faith, I can look past that hurt to share the hope in his heart.

I know that this illness has been merciless and I can only admire John's powerful will. I have seen this determination for many years. Yes, my husband has always been strong, yet I have been privileged to experience other aspects of John's multifaceted personality, many of which first attracted me to him. Because we met at a crucial time in my life when I was hurting inside, I did not believe that I could love again. But John had a strong and gentle way about him that captivated me. I didn't even want to trust him, let alone lose myself in those eyes. Yet there was an intensely exciting, spiritual quality that surrounded John and I was drawn to him like a moth to the flame. He was my magnificent obsession…I guess you could say that John had it going on. As good as that was, over the years I have also come to know his integrity and faith.

Those qualities still draw and hold me close. They are the foundation of my devotion and love for John and throughout this assault, those qualities have remained. Nothing can eradicate them, least of all this retched disease. Grace surrounds him as God leads us on to each new day.

Sometimes, when he is feeling really bad, I hear John saying, "It ain't nothing but a thing." That term came from his army days and my understanding is that it's a way to not to give place to pain, fear or any person that might be trying to get in his mind to do him harm. It does seem to help him cope when he walks through the valley days. Oh, but I have confidence because my John is a mountain climbing man.

On those rare occasions when John is truly down, this is where my strength is most tested. I sometimes fail, sneaking off the bathroom to shed tears on my own. But thank God who then furnishes the grace to keep smiling just when I need it the most.

Apparently, to my great surprise, my smile is important to John as well so much that it makes him feel well again. At least, he often tells me, "Your smile lights up the world." That smile, to me, is my declaration of the light of hope that lives in my heart and bares witness upon my face. It is God expressing his grace through me as he leads me on. Hide it under a bushel. NO. I'm going to let it shine. As long as it brings John cheer, I will smile because love never concludes. It just grows more sweet and precious with the passing of time.

APPENDIX

Cards to copy and give out. When someone shows kindness, pass it on!

You're It

I am what I am, working toward what I want to be in the hope that I can bring joy, laughter, and help and show as many people the correct path as I know it through this Journey called life.

God has given me all that I need. Now it is up to me.

Oh…and now you. You're it. Pass it on.

Thanks, John

You're It

I am what I am, working toward what I want to be in the hope that I can bring joy, laughter, and help and show as many people the correct path as I know it through this Journey called life.

God has given me all that I need. Now it is up to me.

Oh…and now you. You're it. Pass it on.

Thanks, John

The Power of Words

What do your words look like? Want to know? Just look in the faces of those around you. Are they happy—interested—longing for you to go on…or do they have that blank expression filled with a lack of interest? Must they defend against the arrows that you have directed their way?

How many nice things have YOU said today?
*I love you…*You look very nice today…You are good…You work hard and I appreciate it…You are doing great…I will do what I can to help you…You do good work…Thank you…I want you to be happy…I appreciate you…by J.W.W.

Keys for Success

Open as many doors for others as you can, and, above all, never lose your sense of direction. By J.W.W.

Thanks, I needed That!

Sometimes, appreciation never makes it from our brain to our mouth to the ears of the ones that we appreciate. Thanks, I needed that and I DO appreciate you.

Thanks, I needed That!

Sometimes, appreciation never makes it from our brain to our mouth to the ears of the ones that we appreciate. Thanks, I needed that and I DO appreciate you.

Thanks, I needed That!

Sometimes, appreciation never makes it from our brain to our mouth to the ears of the ones that we appreciate. Thanks, I needed that and I DO appreciate you.

Where are you Now?

This is irrelevant. It's fact. It's present. You are right here. What counts is how many people you help or bring along with you. How many people are better because you are here? Most important where are you going…not what have you been or where you are now? By J.W.W

978-0-595-40611-
0-595-40611-4